The Acid Room

The Psychedelic Trials and Tribulations
of Hollywood Hospital

The Acid Room

The Psychedelic Trials and Tribulations
of Hollywood Hospital

JESSE DONALDSON
AND ERIKA DYCK

Anvil Press • Vancouver

Library and Archives Canada Cataloguing in Publication

Title: The acid room : the psychedelic trials and tribulations of Hollywood Hospital / Jesse Donaldson & Erika Dyck.
Names: Donaldson, Jesse, 1982- author. | Dyck, Erika, 1975- author.
Description: Includes bibliographical references.
Identifiers: Canadiana 20210378247 | ISBN 9781772141863 (softcover)
Subjects: LCSH: Hollywood Hospital (New Westminster, B.C.)—History—20th century. | LCSH: Hospitals—British Columbia—New Westminster—History—20th century. | LCSH: LSD (Drug)—Therapeutic use—British Columbia—New Westminster—History—20th century.
Classification: LCC RC483.5.L9 D66 2021 | DDC 616.89/18—dc23
Classification: LCC FC3847.26.F64 D66 2020 | DDC 971.1/3304092—dc23

Book design by Clint Hutzulak/Rayola.com
Represented in Canada by Publishers Group Canada
Distributed by Raincoast Books

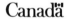 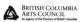

The publisher gratefully acknowledges the financial assistance of the Canada Council for the Arts, the Canada Book Fund, and the Province of British Columbia through the BC Arts Council and the Book Publishing Tax Credit.

Anvil Press Publishers Inc.
PO Box 3008, Station Terminal
Vancouver, BC V6B 3X5 Canada
anvilpress.com

Printed and bound in Canada

"He who is about to come to life under the impact of LSD-25 must first learn how to die.

**— Ben Metcalfe, *Vancouver Province*,
September 1, 1959**

CONTENTS

INTRO (SPEAK TO ME)

If you're hoping for a balanced look at the history of psychedelic drugs in Canada, this book may not be for you.

Discussions of drug use and/or drug policy are rarely balanced; most conversations on the topic are fuelled by emotion — fear, passion, frustration. Those who experiment with illegal drugs are often vilified, or associated with all manner of negative attributes: hedonism, laziness, lack of self-control, addiction. But for the hundreds of patients who visited New Westminster's Hollywood Hospital for legal LSD therapy between 1957 and 1968, the experience wasn't negative at all.

It was life-changing.

Many quit drinking. Others pulled themselves up out of poverty. Some fixed their marriages, or came to terms with lifelong trauma or repressed truths about themselves. A handful kept in touch with their therapists for years afterward. In the majority of cases, patients who underwent psychedelic therapy considered it one of the most useful and meaningful experiences of their entire lives. These are the perspectives generally missing from the "balanced" conversation, and they form the bulk of the narrative contained here.

The Lower Mainland of British Columbia occupies a unique position in the history of global drug policy. Historically, it has been a focal point for research and discussion on the use of illicit drugs; it was home to many of Canada's early psychedelic pioneers, including J. Ross MacLean and Al Hubbard, and the birthplace of InSite, the world's first supervised injection site.

It's also the birthplace of drug prohibition — not just in Canada, but everywhere.

Prior to 1907, drug use in western society was viewed as a personal issue rather than a moral one, and drugs like opium and heroin could be purchased with a doctor's prescription from any corner drugstore. But in the wake of Vancouver's racially motivated anti-Asian riot, in which a white mob destroyed portions of Chinatown, future Prime Minister William Lyon Mackenzie King (then Minister of Labour) was dispatched to survey the damage. Walking the streets, he noticed, to his horror, that Chinatown's opium dens were being frequented by both white and Asian customers. Mackenzie King's worry was race-mixing, not addiction, and in his panicked report to the federal government, he recommended an immediate ban on the smoked opium popular with Chinese Canadians (the injectable version preferred by white Canadians remained legal). This ban was enacted in 1908, and over the next several years, laws prohibiting other narcotic substances appeared across Canada and the United States — all of them racially motivated. Ultimately, the history of drugs in western society is the history of moral panic, racism, and social control. In this, psychedelic drugs are no different; their prohibition stems from a decision by the government of then president Richard Nixon, who sought a cudgel to wield against his main antagonists: African Americans and hippies. As domestic policy chief John Ehrlichman explained, in a 1994 interview with *Harper's* writer Dan Baum, the

Nixon administration "had two enemies: the antiwar left and black people [...] We knew we couldn't make it illegal to be either against the war or black, but by getting the public to associate the hippies with marijuana and blacks with heroin, and then criminalizing both heavily, we could disrupt those communities. We could arrest their leaders, raid their homes, break up their meetings, and vilify them night after night on the evening news. Did we know we were lying about the drugs? Of course we did."

Caught in the middle of this tumultuous moment in history was Hollywood Hospital. It offered legal psychedelic treatments on the eve of the war on drugs, and the stories of recovery coming from within added valuable data to the emerging field of psychedelic science. For a few brief years, it represented a different kind of experimental space: one that flirted with new ideas about how to treat alcoholism, and one that questioned the then-psychiatric (and criminal) diagnosis of homosexuality with insights about love, acceptance, and self-worth. It was a place filled with colourful characters — patients, staff, and a few who blended those roles. Some, like Al Hubbard and Frank Ogden, serve as unreliable narrators, their flair for the dramatic (and untrue) making it sometimes difficult to separate fact from fiction. Luckily, the remnants of Hollywood Hospital's patient records — 534 in total — were deposited at the British Columbia Archives in 2015. The files are not complete, and it's unclear what has been lost, removed, or altered. There are some doctors' and nurses' reports, but the largest cohort comes from the patients themselves: each (complete) case includes a patient autobiography, prompted by a series of open-ended questions. There is a detailed "observers report" that follows, in which exact dosages of mescaline and/or LSD are recorded, along with any developments in the course of the ten-hour (or sometimes longer) observation period — including musical selections and patient responses. The next day, on a blue notepad, subjects recorded their own personal reflections about the experience — often in vivid detail. Despite lurid tabloid claims, the vast majority of patients treated at Hollywood Hospital were not being flown into Vancouver from California. The overwhelming majority were ordinary people, drawn directly from Vancouver and surrounding areas (that said, a handful of patients did come from farther afield, including San Francisco, Hawaii, and as far away as Mexico, Peru, and France). The files are often incredibly candid personal accounts that illustrate how ordinary people contributed to this extraordinary story.

It's fitting in many ways that this book is the result of a collaboration between two authors — one on the West Coast and the other on the Prairies. The history of psychedelic psychiatry itself is a story of collaboration among researchers in Saskatoon and New Westminster, as they attempted to challenge orthodox ways of thinking about mental illness and addiction. We embarked upon this book, from our homes in BC and Saskatchewan, in that same spirit.

And the timing was fortuitous; in recent years, western nations have been undergoing a psychedelic renaissance, and Canada has stepped back into the leading role it held more than fifty years ago. That psychedelic drug use (particularly in controlled environments, or in the company of experienced psychonauts) is beneficial to mental health has, for decades, been beyond debate. Since research began in the 1940s, serious scientists have known that psychedelics in general, and LSD in particular, are among the safest "illicit" substances on earth; they carry no potential for addiction, and little risk of overdose. Medical professionals attest to their usefulness in a psychiatric setting, and the transformative effects of a single experience have been attested to by celebrities and business moguls like Carrie Fisher, Steve Jobs, Sting, Seth Rogen, Angelina Jolie, Anthony Bourdain, Bill Gates, and Susan Sarandon. The hyperbolic media depictions of acid flashbacks and brain damage perpetuated during the 1960s and '70s have proven to be little more than scaremongering, and the positive effects of LSD and psilocybin — even weeks or months after their use — are well documented in dozens of peer-reviewed, academic studies. This book takes those assertions as the well-documented facts that they are.

At the same time, this book is intended to offer more than another historical account of a misunderstood psychedelic clinic; our hope is to provide a window onto some of Canada's earliest discussions about harm reduction and drug regulation, in a region that served as ground zero for both. It is an attempt to provide a counterpoint to the fear and zeal implicit in most conversations about drug use, and to illustrate the critical role Vancouver and New Westminster played in the advancement of psychedelic therapy — one it plays again today. It's intended to give a candid look at the real people whose lives were affected by this unique and maligned form of therapy, and to promote a different way of thinking about addiction, medicine, psychiatry, and the substances we've labelled "illicit." After decades of scaremongering and prohibition, this may not exactly constitute balance.

But it's a start.

At ground zero,
Erika Dyck and Jesse Donaldson
January 2022

Royal Vancouver Yacht Club
1953

The dining room of the Vancouver Yacht Club was an unusual place for a drug deal.

Then again, it was an unusual deal. It was lunchtime, and Dr. Humphry Osmond was seated at a table inside the stately white Jericho Beach clubhouse, surrounded by the city's upper crust. For an instant, he felt intimidated.

"It was a very dignified place," he later recalled, "and I was rather awed by it."

The club was in its golden jubilee year, and things were changing fast.

Members had recently voted to allow powerboats into their fleet — still docked at Coal Harbour, alongside the club's flagship, the *Gometra*. Jayes, the long-time head steward, had retired only a few years earlier, leaving the dining room in the hands of new head steward Frank Cavaliero, who capably managed diners and made space in the discreet upstairs room reserved for members who had imbibed too much.

Apart from feeling out of place, Osmond had no need to be nervous. The deal would attract no attention, even among the city's elite, because the drugs he had come to discuss were legal. Osmond was a researcher — one of the most promising in the country, conducting experiments on mental health and addiction with the blessing of legendary Saskatchewan premier Tommy Douglas. The man he was there to meet was something of an enigma — a passionate amateur with a small fortune, a private plane, and shadowy government connections, a powerfully built former bootlegger with thinning whitish hair, an impish grin, voracious appetites, and a .45 perpetually strapped to his hip. Throughout his life, he would adopt a variety of nicknames, but to Osmond and his cohort, he came to be known simply as "the Captain."

And the Captain wanted mescaline.

Osmond's work, using the compound to study model psychosis, had been much discussed in scholarly circles, and the Captain, an enthusiastic reader of scientific literature, knew that the researcher was his most likely pipeline to the powerful psychedelic (though Osmond wouldn't invent that term for another three years). The discussion then turned from mescaline to a relatively new psychiatric substance — dubbed "Delysid" by Sandoz, its Swiss manufacturer — of which, the Captain claimed, he had recently become the sole licensed Canadian importer.

Huddled at their table, they would have made an interesting pair — the Captain large and boisterous, with a crewcut and a mischievous twinkle in his eye; Osmond thin, bookish, bespectacled, and in professorial tweed. There is little documentation on the length or substance of the meeting, but by Osmond's account, it was a pleasant one.

"He was also very genial, an excellent host," he later noted —
though not without his peculiarities. "He was," Osmond
chuckled, "interested in all sorts of odd things."

But it served as a beginning of sorts, a meeting that would
foster one of the most innovative and divisive fields of psychiatric study in the twentieth century, and transform a nondescript
suburban clinic into a place that was famous (and infamous) all
over North America. Nestled among the holly trees that inspired
its name, Hollywood Hospital became a mecca for high-profile
politicians, celebrities, and seekers of truth. Over the course of
ten years, the approach pioneered by Osmond, the Captain, and
their contemporaries would change thousands of lives, open up
brave new worlds of inquiry, and allow a generation the opportunity to open wide their doors of perception.

Shortly after that, it would be destroyed.

Beset by powerful forces both inside and out — moral, social,
racial, and economic — their work would be driven underground
for more than fifty years. By then, the word "psychedelic" would
be part of the mainstream lexicon, and Delysid would be making
headlines under a more familiar name: LSD. But the Hollywood
Hospital approach would not be properly studied for decades,
the work of the Captain and his contemporaries sealed in boxes,
unseen by all but a few academics. Their approach was simple,
but effective — a comfortable couch, a patterned carpet, an
Impressionist painting, a record player, a vase of flowers, and a
crystal chalice filled with one of the most powerful psychoactive
compounds ever created.

It became known as the Acid Room, and within its walls, patients
would embark on the most meaningful journey of their lives.

Part I: An Inner Restlessness

Fabulous animals move across the scene. Everything is novel and amazing. Almost never does the visionary see anything that reminds him of his own past. He is not remembering scenes, persons, or objects, and he is not inventing them; he is looking on at a new creation.

— Aldous Huxley, *Heaven and Hell*

1
BREATHE

*At other times I danced, stomped, pounded,
sang, turned over a chair, etc. [...] Later on I
thought of people I had felt contempt for before
and realized how unforgiving and callous I had
been. I cried for them and for myself. [...] At the
moment I don't feel as though I'm recapturing
the emotions of the trip by trying to describe
them. I am sure though that they will come
back to reassure me at time when I need them
especially. I think it is a beginning.*

— David V., Hollywood Hospital patient, spring 1968

BY THE LATE 1940S, western psychiatry was at a crossroads.
Most often people with mental illness found themselves removed
from society, housed in large custodial hospitals or asylums, with

little hope of recovery. Therapeutic options for mental illness were limited — either Freudian psychodynamic therapies (or "talk therapies") or, for more severe cases, lifetime in an institution. But the introduction of the first psychopharmaceuticals marked a turning point; throughout the 1950s, antidepressant, antipsychotic, and anti-anxiety medications poured onto the market, suddenly giving doctors new ways to manage illness, bringing with them seemingly limitless potential to transform the field of mental health. Eager to capitalize on this pharmaceutical gold rush, the world's major chemical companies raced to discover the next psychiatric wonder drug.

One such company was Sandoz.

Based in Switzerland, the chemical manufacturer had established a pharmaceutical division in the early part of the twentieth century. They had enjoyed some success with a drug used to treat migraine headaches — one that the division's founder, Arthur Stoll, had synthesized from a poisonous mould known as ergot. Commonly found on rye, ergot had been a well-known remedy since the Middle Ages, used by midwives and healers to promote contractions in childbirth, as well as to induce miscarriage. In large enough quantities, it also caused powerful hallucinations. In fact, some modern historians now posit that several historical instances of mass hysteria were the result of ergot poisoning, including the Salem witch trials and the "Great Fear" of revolutionary France. By 1938, Sandoz chemist Albert Hofmann was one of a small team of chemists working alongside Stoll, tasked with resuming the company's research into its effect on migraines and cluster headaches by extracting pure versions of plant-based compounds, including ergotamine.

The work, Stoll warned him, would be difficult. Nonetheless, Hofmann managed to isolate the nucleus common to all ergot alkaloids — lysergic acid — and worked to synthesize dozens of different compounds utilizing the substance. Hofmann's intent was to study their effects on circulation and respiration, and when administered to lab animals, they largely performed as expected. However, Hofmann noted that one particular batch, labelled LSD-25, tended to make the animals restless. Results weren't promising enough to proceed, and the research was discontinued, but Hofmann suspected that there was more to be learned from those early experiments.

"A peculiar presentiment — the feeling that this substance could possess properties other than those established in the first investigations — induced me, five years after the first synthesis, to produce LSD-25 once again," he later wrote, "so that a sample could be given to the pharmacological department for further tests. This was quite unusual; experimental substances, as a rule, were definitely stricken from the research program if once found to be lacking in pharmacological interest."

On April 16, 1943, working alone, Hofmann synthesized a new batch of LSD-25. Owing to Sandoz's notorious stinginess (they had once refused to install fume hoods in the lab on the grounds that it would be too expensive), he made only a small amount, but during the crystallization process, something strange happened.

"I was forced to interrupt my work in the laboratory in the middle of the afternoon and proceed home, being affected by a remarkable restlessness, combined with a slight dizziness," he wrote, in a memo to Stoll. "At home I lay down and sank into a not unpleasant intoxicated-like condition, characterized by an extremely stimulated imagination. In a dreamlike state, with eyes closed (I found the daylight to be unpleasantly glaring), I perceived an uninterrupted stream of fantastic pictures, extraordinary shapes with intense, kaleidoscopic play of colors."

Hofmann was certain these effects were the result of contact with LSD-25. The compound, it seemed, could be absorbed through the skin. And given the relatively small amount he had synthesized, it appeared to be a substance of extraordinary potency.

Three days later, on April 19, he decided to repeat the experiment under more controlled conditions. With lab assistant Susi Ramstein in tow and a journal in hand, he dosed himself with 250 micrograms of LSD-25 and embarked on the world's first acid trip.

"17:00" he wrote in his journal. "Beginning dizziness, feeling of anxiety, visual distortions, symptoms of paralysis, desire to laugh."

Hofmann quickly became overwhelmed by the sensations, and soon he was struggling to speak intelligibly. So intense were the changes in his perception that he was unable to even keep notes; the second and final entry in his journal reads simply: "MOST SEVERE CRISIS."

Managing to mount a bicycle, Hofmann and Ramstein rode home. But his moment of crisis had only begun.

"On the way home, my condition began to assume threatening forms," he wrote afterward. "Everything in my field of vision wavered and was distorted as if seen in a curved mirror. I also had the sensation of being unable to move from the spot. Nevertheless, my assistant later told me that we had traveled very rapidly. Finally, we arrived at home safe and sound, and I was just barely capable of asking my companion to summon our family doctor and request milk from the neighbours."

Convinced he had been poisoned, Hofmann drank two litres of milk, hoping it might negate some of the compound's effects. Hysterical, he asked Ramstein to call for a doctor, and to telephone his wife.

"A demon had invaded me, had taken possession of my body, mind, and soul. I jumped up and screamed, trying to free myself from him, but then sank down again and lay helpless on the sofa. The substance, with which I had wanted to experiment, had vanquished me. It was the demon that scornfully triumphed over my will. I was seized by the dreadful fear of going insane."

Lying on his couch, Hofmann reflected, with "bitter irony: if I was now forced to leave this world prematurely, it was because of this lysergic acid diethylamide that I myself had brought forth into the world."

That he had suffered such an extreme reaction is hardly surprising; unaware of LSD's true potency, Hofmann had consumed roughly two-and-a-half times the amount considered standard by today's researchers. But the doctor could find nothing wrong with Hofmann, apart from dilated pupils. As the hours passed, he settled into the experience, and found himself enjoying the colours and shapes on display. His wife, returning home in a panic, found Hofmann at ease, and able to explain what had happened. He slept the night, and awoke the next morning feeling renewed.

"A sensation of well-being and renewed life flowed through me," he wrote. "Breakfast tasted delicious and gave me extraordinary pleasure. When I later walked out into the garden, in which the sun shone now after a spring rain, everything glistened and sparkled in a fresh light. The world was as if newly created. All my senses vibrated in a condition of highest sensitivity, which persisted for the entire day."

Roughly two months later, his assistant Susi Ramstein had an LSD experience of her own, taking 100 micrograms of LSD and boarding a tram. She would participate in a total of three LSD experiments, and her dosage would ultimately become the standard for medical use.

Hofmann was intrigued by his discovery. But neither he nor Sandoz had the faintest idea what to do with it.

Luckily, there were other researchers who did.

In 1944, Saskatchewan elected the first socialist government in North America.

The province's new premier, Tommy Douglas, had campaigned on promises of reforming the health care system, and over the next twenty years, he and his Co-operative Commonwealth Federation government established the framework for what would ultimately become Canada's national medicare program. As he embarked on those reforms, Douglas readily recognized the need to invest in medical research alongside public policy reforms, working to transform Saskatchewan into a scientific incubator, recruiting the best medical minds in the world to gather and stimulate a culture of experimentation.

One such recruit was Humphry Osmond.

Feeling stifled by the overly bureaucratic environment of British medicine, the English psychiatrist moved from London to Saskatchewan in 1951, to take a position as the clinical director of the Saskatchewan Mental Hospital at Weyburn.

When Osmond arrived, he was horrified by what he saw.

The hospital itself maintained an impressive exterior and meticulously manicured gardens, but beyond the façade, patients suffered, administrators were embroiled in scandal, and staff were more often chosen through patronage than skill.

"It looks as if the current mental hospitals are the worst possible for schizophrenic people," he lamented in a letter. "They are unsuitable for human habitation and are especially bad for sick humans, particularly those with perceptual disorders. Sometimes I wilt beneath the follies."

He would refer to the gigantic hospital (by some estimates the largest in the British Commonwealth) as the "Augean stables," referring to the unholy mess tackled during the fifth labour of Hercules. Luckily, within weeks of arriving in Saskatchewan, Osmond met someone who would become a partner in those labours: fellow psychiatrist and biochemist Abram Hoffer. Hoffer had grown up in Saskatchewan and had recently returned to take up a research position at the University of

Saskatchewan's new medical school in Saskatoon. Osmond and Hoffer became close collaborators; despite the hundreds of miles that separated them geographically, they were connected by a desire to improve mental health care and support provincial health care reforms — with a particular focus on hallucinations and psychosis.

Osmond knew that psychotic disorders, like schizophrenia, were the most prevalent forms of mental illness in most asylums, and that historically, there were no clinical options for patients beyond rest and confinement. But the pharmaceutical revolution provided new opportunities for study, and two compounds quickly caught his eye: mescaline and LSD-25. Osmond's early work had focused on the idea of "model psychosis," chemically induced neurological changes that could allow clinicians to personally experience the schizophrenic mind. LSD and mescaline, he theorized, could mimic the psychotic effects of schizophrenia, and by producing such a model of a disease, doctors could better empathize with patients. Indeed, some referred to these drugs as "psychotomimetic" for their alleged ability to induce illness-like states. It was believed that self-experimentation with these substances would allow physicians, nurses, and social workers to gain valuable insight into the plight of their patients by giving them a temporary excursion into madness.

In the beginning, these theories were tested through self-experimentation. Many of Osmond and Hoffer's early medical explorations took place in the comfort of their own living rooms. The pair often participated in these home experiments themselves — sometimes alone, sometimes in the company of friends and spouses.

In addition to their work with model psychosis, Hoffer and Osmond began exploring LSD and mescaline to treat alcoholics. They hypothesized that an LSD experience could mirror the terrifying descriptions of "hitting rock bottom" regularly described by alcoholic patients. Those suffering from alcoholism often rejected help until reaching that stage (a point confirmed by Alcoholics

Anonymous). Osmond and Hoffer reasoned that by giving alcoholics a dose of LSD, they could hijack the natural course of the
disease by artificially inducing the "rock bottom" state, and consequently avoid the physiological and physical damage wrought by
long-term, problem drinking. Early results were promising. They
began publishing in medical journals, and their research attracted
significant attention. For the first time since LSD's synthesis in 1938,
the field of psychedelic study was finally being given room to
breathe, and some of the most significant research in the world was
being conducted in Canada.

Their work was also attracting attention outside scientific circles.

In March 1953, Osmond received a letter from *Brave New World*
author Aldous Huxley. Huxley had learned of his research program,
and, fascinated by the possibilities, requested an opportunity to
experience mescaline for himself. With the compound in hand,
Osmond drove to Los Angeles to meet Aldous and Maria Huxley,
and their meeting quickly cemented a friendship that would last
until Huxley's death in 1963. And it was through Huxley that
Osmond and Hoffer met the man destined to play a significant role
in the evolution of psychedelic psychiatry, a man who would serve as
both hero and villain in the years ahead.

His name was Al Hubbard, but to them, he would become
known simply as "the Captain."

2

ON THE RUN

Life is an eternal try — this life, any life, every life. And we all have choice — millions and millions of big and little choices. Decisions! Decisions. And we won't make them all right — but we won't make them all wrong.

— Kelly S., Hollywood Hospital patient, spring 1962

THERE IS PERHAPS NO BETTER AVATAR for the drug he helped popularize than Alfred M. Hubbard.

To anyone who made his acquaintance, he seemed a strange mix of fact and fiction, a mass of contradictory elements; impish, yet imposing. Religious, yet unscrupulous. Conservative, yet open to experimentation with all manner of psychotropic substances. Born in rural Kentucky to an alcoholic father, he likely left school at a young age, moving west to settle in Washington state. While formally uneducated, he possessed a keen intellect that was matched only by a flamboyant streak and a willingness to play fast and loose with the facts. A devout Catholic, he told friends that, during his preteen years, he had been visited by an angel who encouraged him to pursue science. It was this heavenly visitor, he said, that led to the invention of a device he dubbed the "atmospheric energy generator." A July 1920 issue of the *Seattle Post-Intelligencer* reported on the invention, alongside "boy inventor" Hubbard's claims that it could provide limitless power, pulled directly from the "cosmic energy" in the air. Hubbard even staged a demonstration, using the device to power an eighteen-foot boat around Lake Union.

"The inventor says that so far as he has been able to learn, its life as a power unit is indefinite," reported the paper breathlessly. "He declared that a coil large enough to drive an airplane would be no more than three times the size of the coil used yesterday, and that a machine thus equipped could fly around the world without stopping, so far as the power supply is concerned."

Whether the device actually performed as advertised is, like many of Hubbard's boasts, suspect. Claiming he was awaiting a patent, he kept engineers from inspecting it, and when interest quickly faded, Hubbard snatched up his investors' money and disappeared.

In the fall of 1920, when he was barely twenty, he married his sixteen-year-old neighbour, May Cunningham. A likely reason for the marriage was that Cunningham was already pregnant, and the pair moved into a small apartment, barely making ends meet, as Hubbard dodged creditors and tried to keep out of sight. After the furor died down, he opened a small radio shop in Seattle — which is how he came to the attention of legendary Puget Sound bootlegger Roy Olmstead. A former cop, Olmstead had become a kingpin during Prohibition, reportedly the single biggest employer in the region. For years, Olmstead had the local police in his pocket, but now federal prohibition agents were beginning to sniff around, and he needed a handful of new tricks to stay out of prison. Having read of Hubbard's scientific exploits in local papers, Olmstead asked the former boy inventor to furnish him with sophisticated radio equipment that would allow his fleet of boats, planes, and cars to keep one step ahead of the government.

True to form, Hubbard extracted a long list of concessions: Olmstead paid his outstanding debts, gave him a car, allowed him to move into the basement of the liquor kingpin's lavish estate (with its own lab), and gave Hubbard's wife an expense account. In return, Hubbard became Olmstead's tech wizard. He kept the bootlegger's fleet of vehicles in working order, and installed sophisticated, long-range ship-to-shore radio equipment. At the advice of Olmstead's wife, they eventually built a full-fledged radio station (KFQX) in October 1924, using it as a legitimate business through which to funnel money. Over time, Hubbard also grew to become one of Olmstead's most trusted lieutenants; he learned the finer points of bootlegging, and attended the lavish parties thrown on Olmstead's estate.

Which made it all the more disappointing that Hubbard was the one to betray him.

By the fall of 1924, federal agents were closing in. They raided Olmstead's property, arresting everyone they could find — including Al Hubbard. At twenty-three years old, he found his reputation in tatters. His finances were in ruins. His young wife filed for divorce. So he did the only thing he could think of: he flipped.

Once again, his skill as a negotiator and his complete lack of scruples paid off; William Whitney, the agent in charge, had Hubbard's name removed from the indictment, and hired him as a prohibition agent. It was an unusual arrangement for the time — but then, Hubbard wasn't much of an agent. He filed very few reports, and those he did file deliberately unhelpful. In the meantime, he continued to pilot ships for Olmstead, delivering booze and evading prohibition agents in the dead of night. The charade wouldn't last.

Arrested during one of his late-night liquor runs, Hubbard found that he had used up all of Whitney's goodwill; calling Olmstead in for a meeting, the prohibition agent revealed that Hubbard had been playing both sides, and the bootlegger soon found himself in front of a judge.

"Well, Roy — the jig is up," Whitney said. "Hubbard is an agent and he absolutely has the goods on you and a lot more others."

"Well, I'll be damned," Olmstead replied, stunned. "I never would have believed it. That damn scoundrel certainly fooled me good."

After hesitating for a few moments, he simply concluded, "Well, I'm done."

Incredibly, Hubbard remained in Olmstead's employ. As the booze magnate prepared for his day in court, Hubbard convinced his boss that he was mining the department for inside info — a performance that proved so convincing that Olmstead even paid Hubbard protection money. At the same time, Hubbard would inform Whitney's department about upcoming alcohol shipments, before turning around and warning Olmstead's bootleggers about the impending raids.

By 1927, he was on thin ice.

After working in several different jurisdictions, he convinced the bureau that he was the man to infiltrate a smuggling ring in Vancouver, BC. Once a part of their ranks, he turned on the government, telling the bootleggers that they could pay him for protection from the coast guard — and what's more, he would guarantee the shipment personally.

It didn't go as planned.

The smugglers they met on the open water recognized Hubbard as a federal agent and opened fire. Hubbard pulled his pistol and somehow gained the upper hand, handcuffing the crew to the deck and bringing the boat to shore, where they were arrested.

In the resulting media storm, Hubbard's corruption was revealed. An investigation ensued, and he was terminated from the department in September 1927. A month later, he was the star witness at Roy Olmstead's trial. Hubbard held nothing back, and Olmstead was found guilty on all charges. Even though he had publicly betrayed a major figure in the criminal underworld, Hubbard not only avoided retribution, but managed to continue working as a bootlegger. And despite his unceremonious dismissal, he kept in touch with William Whitney, in hopes of one day being reinstated as a prohibition agent. But Whitney had no intention of allowing the traitorous Hubbard back into the ranks — something he made abundantly clear when the pair met in a hallway at bureau headquarters in Seattle.

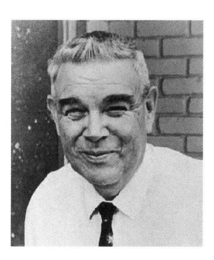

Captain Al Hubbard.

"I want you to go away and stay away," Whitney shouted. "What you ought to do is go back to your radio business and make a success of it and give up on the idea that you can ever get back on the force."

Hubbard was furious — so furious that he began a campaign of misinformation about Whitney and his involvement with the Seattle underworld. The evidence, though flimsy, was enough to warrant a trial, and even though it resulted in a not-guilty verdict, Whitney was ultimately dismissed from his job.

In the ensuing years, Hubbard went back to working with radio technology. But it wouldn't last; he soon returned to his old ways. On a rum-running excursion, he met a woman named Rita, and the pair later got married. By 1936, he was again playing both sides of the law, working as a temporary prohibition agent outside Seattle, while simultaneously assisting millionaire bootlegger Johnny Marino. This time, however, his luck ran out; he was arrested, and spent two years in McNeil Island Penitentiary.

Following his release, Hubbard decided he no longer wanted to live his life on the run. He obtained his master-of-sea-vessels certification, and became Captain Hubbard, skipper of a luxury yacht. When World War II broke out, he was approached by the government to smuggle military supplies back and forth across the US–Canadian border. Hubbard and Rita moved their family north, opening a front business in Vancouver called Marine Sales and Service, with Hubbard installed as "director of engineering." During the war years, he became fabulously wealthy; in addition to Marine Sales and Service, he also started a company that dealt in nuclear materials. By the end of the war, he owned a yacht called the *Misenderan*, a fleet of aircraft, and Dayman Island, a 24-acre chunk of land four miles off the coast of Vancouver Island. He had, it seemed, left his criminal past behind. But Hubbard was restless.

"Al was desperately searching for meaning in his life," explained long-time friend Willis Harman.

In 1952, seeking enlightenment, he returned to an area near Spokane, Washington, where he'd spent summers during his youth. And it was there, in a clearing, that he received his second angelic vision.

"She [the angel] told Al that something tremendously important to the future of mankind would be coming soon, and that he could play a role in it if he wanted to," Harman noted. "But he hadn't the faintest clue what he was supposed to be looking for."

It would become clear soon enough.

Meanwhile, Aldous Huxley had just undertaken his first mescaline trip, and it changed everything. Despite Osmond's misgivings that he risked going down in history as "the man who drove Aldous Huxley mad," the experience had inspired the author to express himself in writing, and had also opened his mind to new connections — connections Huxley wove together into a book he titled *The Doors of Perception*. By the time Huxley's slim volume reached bookshelves, the psychedelic cat was out of the bag. It wasn't long before Al Hubbard, a voracious reader, heard about the experience and wanted to see it for himself. Hubbard had his first mescaline trip on Dayman Island and, for him, as for Huxley, it was a transformative moment.

"It was the deepest mystical thing I've ever seen," he later wrote. "I saw myself as a tiny mite in a big swamp with a spark of intelligence. I saw my mother and father having intercourse. It was all clear."

And now, after years of searching for meaning, Hubbard felt as though he had found his calling, the elusive *something* outlined in his angelic vision that could change the world. Leafing through a copy of *The Hibbert Journal*, Hubbard noted the work of British psychiatrist Humphry Osmond, who wrote about mescaline's ability to connect medicine, philosophy, and spirituality. And shortly after that, he came across LSD-25. He was an instant convert. He flew to London and managed to secure a whopping forty-three cases of the compound (which proved a challenge for customs), bringing them to Dayman Island to begin his own experiments.

Alongside his wife Rita and an expanding group of friends, he familiarized himself with the drug's effects, outfitting a hangar on the property with art and music (including Gabriel Max's optical-illusion painting *Jesus Christas*) to enhance the experience. Now Al Hubbard had become a different sort of captain — not of luxury yachts or private planes, but of the mind.

However, his adventures with LSD left him craving steady supplies. Remembering Osmond's name from *The Hibbert Journal*, he reached out to the psychiatrist, and in 1953 the pair sat down for lunch at the Vancouver Yacht Club. The meeting left an impression on Osmond, and despite the difference in their backgrounds, both he and Huxley readily took to the Captain. They recognized his manner was coarser than theirs, but they also saw in Hubbard a dreamer and a man of action. Plus, Hubbard's unabashed pursuit of funds and broad network of contacts made him an intriguing collaborator.

"Hubbard is a terrific man of action," Huxley wrote in 1954, "and results of his efforts may begin appearing quite soon."

"He wants to help and I think is likely to do so because he looks upon his function as providing and seeing that money is provided," Osmond wrote, "and not directing how it shall be used. He is in a position to help, having many well placed and well to do friends in both [the] U.S. and Canada, including Nelson Rockefeller who is apparently the most active of the old tycoon's spawn."

Initially, Osmond saw Hubbard's role as more of an investor than a scientist or therapist, noting that his intended function was "quartermaster, not staff officer." But their impression of the Captain quickly softened — in no small part thanks to Hubbard's notorious charm and ambition.

"So glad you like the Captain," Osmond wrote to Huxley. "I felt he was the sort of man we need. I wish he would come and be my business manager here. [...] He is just cut out to get these projects going. The practical man to all outward appearances but with a fine sense of adventure."

Shortly afterward, Osmond encouraged Hubbard to connect with Abram Hoffer. Hubbard didn't skip a beat. A licensed MD with legal access to hallucinogenic drugs, Hoffer was an important connection, and he welcomed Al Hubbard with open arms.

"I think that you are carrying on some very useful and bold experimentation regarding the use of the hallucinogenic compounds," Hoffer enthused in a letter. "I hope that you will continue this work, as it will lead to some very important new principles in the field of psychiatry and general medicine."

Before long, Hubbard was a member of their inner circle, and something of an acid expert. Duncan Blewett, a psychologist working with Osmond in Saskatchewan, later claimed that although Hubbard did not have medical training, "he knew more about acid in his little finger than most of us did."

He continued experimenting, soon incorporating a mixture of carbon dioxide and oxygen known as carbogen, which he kept in portable tanks stashed all over Dayman Island.

"He showed up for lunch one afternoon, and he brought with him a portable tank filled with a gas of some kind," Maria Huxley once recalled. "He offered some to us, but we said we didn't care for any, so he put it down and we all had lunch. He went into the bathroom with the tank after lunch and breathed into it for about ten seconds. It must have been very concentrated, because he came out revitalized and very jubilant, talking about a vision he had seen of the Virgin Mary."

Hubbard also managed to bring in new supplies and chase down new opportunities. But, not content simply to join the inner circle, he wanted to define it; in 1956, he founded the Commission for the Study of Creative Imagination (CSCI), designing an elaborate letterhead with a kaleidoscopic symbol, and a cross in its centre, surrounded by crystalline geometric designs. Declaring himself the scientific director, he peppered his letterhead with the names of influential thinkers, including Osmond, Hoffer, UN technical assistance director Hugh Keenleyside, and Huxley's close friend, the philosopher Gerald Heard. It's unclear if the CSCI had any formal function, or was simply more Hubbard bluster, but it did cement relationships that would stimulate an exciting period of experimentation. Expanding on his previous work on Dayman Island, he tinkered with various parameters — number of participants, inclusion of artwork and lighting — in hopes of perfecting the method.

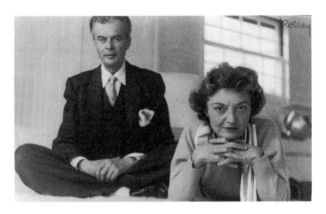

Aldous and Laura Huxley. Undated image.

In particular, the Captain's work with lighting during psychedelic sessions had dazzling results, which left Osmond and others scrambling to find a scientific justification for the perceptual changes.

"And, talking of lanterns — did I tell you that my friend Dr Cholden had found that the stroboscope improved on mescalin effects, just as Al Hubbard did?" Huxley wrote to Osmond. "His own geometrical visions turned, under the flashing lamp, to Japanese landscapes. How the hell this fits in with the notion that stroboscopic effects result from the interference of two rhythms, the lamp's and the brain waves', I cannot imagine."

And even though he wasn't always successful, Hubbard remained focused on a key facet of Osmond and Hoffer's work: using psychedelic therapy to confront past trauma.

"Your nice Captain tried a new experiment," Huxley wrote to Osmond about a session in early 1955, "group mescalinization. It worked very well for Gerald and myself, hardly at all for Bill Forthman, who was given a small dose (200 mmg to our 300) and who had a subconscious resistance of tremendous power, and rather poorly for Hubbard, who tried to run the group in the way he had run other groups in Vancouver, where the drug has worked as a device for raising buried guilts and traumas and permitting people to get on to better terms with themselves."

At the same time, Hubbard's bold approach to networking soon became legendary — though, as was often the case, it tended toward more hype than reality.

"I am hopeful that the good Captain, whose connections with Uranium seem to serve as a passport into the most exalted spheres of government, business and ecclesiastical polity, is about to take off for New York, where I hope he will storm the United Nations, take Nelson Rockefeller for a ride to Heaven and return with millions of dollars," gushed Aldous Huxley in a letter. "What Babes in the Wood we literary gents and professional men are! The great World occasionally requires your services, is mildly amused by mine; but its full attention and deference are paid to Uranium and Big Business. So what extraordinary luck that this representative of both these Higher Powers should (a) have become so passionately interested in mescalin and (b) be such a very nice man."

Hubbard spent much of 1955 and 1956 on the move, spreading the gospel of hallucinogens and working to obtain both supplies and money. On Christmas Eve 1955, he took Huxley on his first acid trip. After that, he flew to Colorado, and oversaw an LSD session with a wealthy, older woman that demonstrated the money-making potential of his work.

"She is seventy-two years old and has had a great deal of trouble during her entire lifetime due to forgotten incidents in her childhood which she had succeeded in repressing from conscious memory," Hubbard wrote in a letter. "Under LSD, we easily brought the incident she feared most to light. After the LSD session, during which she almost went frantic with fear, her character change was most pronounced and she was one of the most delighted persons you ever saw[...]I have several letters from her, and she has several friends now with troubles who would like to try out the idea themselves, offering to pay all expenses and so forth."

By now, researchers had identified that mescaline and LSD seemed to hold the greatest therapeutic potential, so Hubbard made several more stops in search of supplies, before landing in California to meet with Kenneth Ericson of Sandoz, who "complimented us most highly on our little Commission, its high level of operation and excellent results." Hubbard, never one to squander an opportunity, undoubtedly pressed Ericson for supplies and further intel. Hoping to foster his own local supply chain, he also met with scientists at West Coast–based Ampex Laboratories, and urged them to consider working with LSD.

Hubbard was undeterred by laws, supply lines, or anything else that might stand in his way. By the mid-1950s, mescaline was illegal in California. But Hubbard, ever the drug enforcement agent, met with the head of the California Narcotic Enforcement division, and used his powers of persuasion to convince him to ask "the Attorney General of California for a clearance for our work, and I have no doubt we will receive it without trouble."

Hubbard's other main obstacle to obtaining a ready supply of LSD and mescaline was his lack of academic credentials. So, in typical Hubbard fashion, he went out and purchased them, buying a PhD in biopsychology from a less-than-reputable diploma mill known as Taylor University.

"Congratulations on having your PhD," Hoffer wrote in early 1956. "I know you will agree with me when I say that the absence or presence of a PhD means little regarding the ability of an individual to investigate nature's phenomena. It is, however, a recognition that the individual has gone through a prescribed training in scientific investigation and which also provides him with a certain amount of society approval which permits him to carry on his work more readily."

Privately, however, Hubbard's academic colleagues were less impressed by his desire to cut corners.

"The fact that he did not have to attend a University for it makes it the more precious," complained Osmond. "In Al's world, wise men buy cheap and sell, well a trifle less cheaply. As he sees it the acquisition of the fireman's hat is just a transaction of that sort. Only stuffed shirts would see anything wrong about this. Al believes that little difficulties of this sort can always be fixed with a bit of dexterity. And so they sometimes can when the business man bears rich enough gifts to seduce the academic strumpet. But she is a bit choosey these days and Al has not equipped himself with enough cash for the job. So Al has now got to recognise that the scientific and business worlds have their rules and customs, and that one would be well advised to enquire how one differs from the other before jumping out of one into the other."

"His methods of exposition are a bit muddled," Huxley agreed, "but I suppose he and his group have by now a mass of written material on their cases — material which will show how the other line of experimentation works. For obviously one must proceed on both lines — the pure-scientific, analytical line of Puharich [Henry Puharich, American parapsychological researcher] trying out factor after factor in a standardized environment, and the line of the naturalist, psychologist and therapist, who uses the drug for healing and enlightening, and in the process, if he is a good observer and clear thinker, discovers new facts about the psycho-physical organism."

While Hubbard and others had marvelled at how mescaline helped to uncover repressed traumas, he then turned his attention to an old standby from his days as a prohibition agent: alcohol.

"I'd been told by my friend, Captain Hubbard, that people treated by this method were able to drink socially," Osmond explained to David Lester at Yale University.

Osmond confessed to holding much more "orthodox" views when it came to problem drinking — that abstinence was the only solution. But Hubbard challenged this conventional attitude when he showed Osmond that there were other options.

"Under the influence of LSD or mescalin [sic] the person can begin to review themselves and if this is pursued determinedly, they can begin to alter themselves," he wrote. He travelled to California to see Hubbard in action.

Upon his return, Osmond described meeting a pilot who, after 15,000 hours of flying experience, had plummeted to a life on the streets of Vancouver, consuming up to three bottles of whisky a day. Friends considered him dead. He rejected help of any kind.

"It was in this condition that my friend, Captain Hubbard met him," Osmond wrote, "and I think with extraordinary courage, administered mescalin to him."

By the time the pilot met with Osmond, he had transformed his life. He got his old job back, and even made enough money to make some investments and drive "the largest Cadillac that I've ever driven in."

"However, that isn't the most remarkable thing," Osmond continued. Even more notable than bouncing back from rock bottom was the fact that the pilot was able to drink socially after his LSD treatments. "I understand from my friend that he drinks socially and moderately and has never shown the least sign of backsliding," he said, incredulous. "I think you will agree that this is the strangest thing of all about it. Whether other people can reproduce results of this sort I don't know. [...] I think that perhaps we have the beginnings of an enormously potent therapeutic weapon".

From Osmond's perspective, there was only one thing missing: a name — a brand-new word to quantify the brand-new class of drug they were working with, and the experience it provided. In April 1956, he confided to Hoffer that he wanted something specific. It shouldn't, he said, connote madness — the drugs didn't "mimic" psychosis — or signal any particular branch of psychiatry or science. Hoffer, Osmond, and Huxley had been discussing the idea at length, but had thus far been unable to settle on an appropriate term. Contenders at the time included "phantastica," "psychomimetic," and "psychorhexic." Huxley suggested "panerotheyme," jotting down a couplet in a letter to Osmond:

To make this mundane world sublime,
Just half a gram of panerotheyme.

Later that same month, Osmond replied with a couplet of his own:

To plumb the depths or soar angelic,
You'll need a pinch of psychedelic.

The psychedelic era had begun.

By the end of 1956, Al Hubbard moved the commission's head-quarters to a former brothel at 500 Alexander Street, in a decidedly downmarket part of town. His search for money and supplies continued, but at the same time, an idea had taken root in his head. His work with alcoholism and repressed trauma was proving highly effective, and was attracting all the right kinds of attention. The time had come to expand his operation.

And he already had his sights set on just such a setting.

3

TIME

I felt my old self having completely fallen away from me, with almost no recollection of what it was like before. I wanted to get up and take the wax off and 'be' in the world as in the LSD experience. I felt totally loving, accepting, understanding, one with nature and the universe.

— Hilary A., Hollywood Hospital patient, summer 1958

HOLLYWOOD HOSPITAL WAS, in many ways, an unlikely destination for Hubbard to set up shop.

Located at 525 Sixth Street, New Westminster, it was far from the burgeoning psychedelic scene. In fact, the fifty-five-bed facility had been in operation since 1919. Originally established as a tuberculosis

sanitorium, it came under new direction in 1956 when it was purchased by Dr. John Ross MacLean.

"MacLean was tall, handsome, well dressed," noted *Province*
reporter Ben Metcalfe, "a smooth mixture of business and medicine."

Raised in upscale Kerrisdale, the dark-haired, moustached Mac-
Lean had joined Hollywood Hospital's staff in 1954, after completing
his medical training in Manitoba, and went on to purchase the facility when its previous superintendent, Dr. E. A. Campbell, died
suddenly in a boating accident. Luckily, a "smooth mixture of business and medicine" was precisely what the hospital needed; deeply
religious, unfailingly optimistic, and firmly community-minded,
MacLean kept Campbell's widow on the payroll as a receptionist, and
got to work turning the facility's fortunes around.

When MacLean took over as director, the field of alcohol studies
was languishing.

The client files littering his desk were a mess of overdue payments
and third-party payment plans. Another folder was filled with direc-
tives from veterans' organizations, seeking advice on reducing costs,
without necessarily authorizing sufficient treatment. As in other
addiction treatment centres in the 1950s, the medical options were
limited. MacLean inherited a program that relied on a non-stan-
dardized blend of electric shock therapy, psychotherapy, group
therapy, and some crude pharmacological options — sedatives, anti-
psychotics, and a drug known by the trade name Antabuse, designed
to alter the taste of alcohol so that consumers developed an aversion.
In the days before Canada's socialized medicine scheme, the combination of treatments depended as much on payment programs as on
therapeutic rationales. Many clients returned for multiple sessions
— though most had no choice, forced to log hours by judges, parole
officers, or their pension plans. The hospital's prospects seemed
grim. MacLean could continue to treat patients using standard
(though only moderately effective) methods, and spend his time

chasing down payments, or he could look for more effective options. But MacLean had his own surprisingly progressive theories about harm reduction and addiction — ones that were greatly out of step with the times.

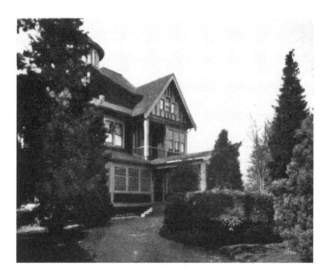

One of the few surviving images of Hollywood Hospital.
Undated photo.

Shortly after graduation, he had taken part in a community pilot project that supplied low-cost drugs to users — in tandem with therapy and skills training — in hopes of lifting them out of poverty. The results were promising: all seven of MacLean's subjects obtained employment. Unfortunately, the project's goals were abruptly changed (against MacLean's wishes) to emphasize abstinence, and every volunteer subsequently returned to life on the street.

In the summer of 1955, MacLean was one of a handful of medical experts arguing before a Senate hearing for the decriminalization of drugs. Addiction, MacLean said, was a mental health concern, and needed to be treated as such.

"They have an incurable disease," he told the Senate, "and if they do not get the narcotics to satisfy their craving legally, they will get them illegally. Proper administration of drugs at cost could keep many addicts in useful work and respectability."

His pleas fell on deaf ears. But when MacLean took over Hollywood Hospital the following year, he sought to use those same ideas to expand the facility's treatment approach.

Which is exactly when he met the Captain.

At first, it seemed an odd combination — MacLean's "smooth mixture of business and medicine" standing in stark contrast to a man Ben Metcalfe later described as a "squat, rumpled, wryly jocular and supremely confident gnostic." Nonetheless, Hubbard's sales pitch impressed MacLean. The director needed a fresh approach to treating alcoholism, and Hubbard's ideas were both novel and dynamic. Hubbard's knowledge of the human condition convinced MacLean to devote an entire wing of the hospital to the study of psychedelic therapy for chronic alcoholics. He even let "Dr." Hubbard run it as the "director of research." It certainly helped that, when it came to Sandoz LSD, Hubbard was now Canada's sole licensed importer.

"How Dr. Hubbard came to be the sole licensed importer of pure Sandoz LSD into Canada and perhaps even the United States, he has never fully explained," wrote Ben Metcalfe years later, "but he was that in those days, and I confirmed it with the Ottawa Food and Drug people."

The time, it seemed, had finally come for psychedelic psychiatry to assume a place of prominence in the world of medicine. So Mac-Lean decided to take a leap of faith.

Little did he know how much faith would be required.

Meanwhile, membership in Hubbard's commission expanded, and its members busied themselves by widening the search for personnel, funds, substances, techniques, and creative influences. Hubbard wrote dozens of letters from the commission's new address at 1308 Powell Street, chasing down a new product known as lysergic acid morpholide. LSM closely resembled Sandoz's LSD, but with a sedative added — leading, in the opinion of Hubbard and Hoffer, to disappointing effects. With Hoffer's background in chemistry and Hubbard's penchant for new chemical combinations, they began to explore alternatives to the traditional Sandoz supply chain.

"I am mailing you today a small bottle containing 25 doses of LSD," Hubbard explained to Hoffer. "This is a new kind of material and is made by a friend of mine in Seattle, who is a research biochemist. Would you please have it mixed with tartaric acid and distilled water, and put into ampules, and mailed back to me here at the hospital as soon as possible, as I want to try it out."

While working to set up the Hollywood Hospital program, Hubbard remained in close contact with his Saskatchewan colleagues.

"We would appreciate your suggestions in setting up a research programme with the Sandos [sic] Company for the hospital," he wrote to Hoffer, emphasizing that both Stanford University and Los Angeles Veterans Hospital were becoming curious about their psychedelic treatments — with dozens of patients now lining up for this option.

As Hubbard and MacLean's preparation continued, they paid particular attention to the physical space in which the sessions would occur. Hubbard knew from personal experience, and from dozens of previous sessions, that comfortable surroundings were key to allaying the anxiety often experienced by patients in the early stages of a drug experience.

But it needed to be about more than comfort; Osmond's early experiments had incorporated spacious rooms and complex artwork, and Hollywood Hospital's psychedelic therapy rooms took this notion even further, providing comfortable couches, patterned rugs, access to a private bathroom, fresh cut flowers, and appropriate music. For Hubbard, the experience yielded the most positive results when it was choreographed and free of outside interruption.

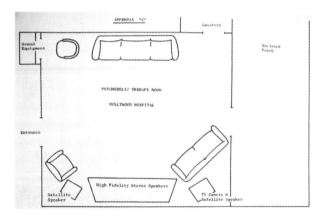

Floor Plan for the Acid Room, circa 1965.

Buoyed by their progress, Hubbard journeyed to Stanford in the middle of 1957, and by all accounts made a good impression on the academic community. But in the weeks that followed, his purchased diploma began to raise eyebrows among serious researchers, and Osmond and Huxley worried that his antics could undermine the movement they were trying to advance.

"Unluckily, instead of using his nautical moniker he [...] paraded himself as Doctor Hubbard," Osmond griped to Huxley. "I feared that he would do this. The result is that his considerable success may be the source of an even greater embarrassment. They wanted to start a sort of LSD research unit and were about to approach the University for some cash. Professor Kumler of the School of Pharmacy looked up Dr H. in *U.S. Men of Science* and he was not there. Very reasonably he feels that it is better for Al's friends to know how much false rigging he is wearing rather than the University Council should discover and brand him an imposter. I have pointed out that he is not a fraud, but an innocent."

There are very few records of patients being treated with LSD or mescaline at Hollywood Hospital in 1957 — likely because the bulk of that time was dedicated to fundraising and experimentation. During this period, many of MacLean and Hubbard's contemporaries — including Dr. Duncan Blewett — were themselves undergoing acid experiences in Saskatchewan to gain a more thorough understanding of the drug and its effects. Hubbard, meanwhile, split his time between counselling patients in New Westminster and travelling the continent in search of money.

"If we can ever really say we have discovered a new aspect of the mind that can do so and so under certain stimuli," he told Hoffer, "than [sic] enormous amounts of money would be immediately available." Furthermore, he said, they could easily raise "a half a million dollars for the research hospital," and offered to organize a financial appeal across Canada.

But, for Hubbard, the financial possibilities were limited if confined to mere scientific inquiry; as far as he could tell, the real money lay in collaborating with the Catholic Church.

"It must be remembered," he told members of the Commission, "although our work has been under medical supervision[...] the problems of an alcoholic are quite different from the orthodox one."

Through his own network, he gathered a number of key players. He was dismayed to learn that there was only one Catholic psychiatrist in Vancouver, so he recruited another from Montreal.

"I was delighted to meet him," Hubbard told the commission, "but he did not seem so enthusiastic towards me." The young Catholic psychiatrist did not understand why the Church should go against its own teachings. "He was quite suspicious of the whole project," Hubbard added, and "couldn't imagine why the Church was involved with it, and why a non-medical man was allowed to tamper with drugs."

Despite his hesitations, the psychiatrist reluctantly agreed to undergo his own LSD session, accompanied by Hubbard, two members of the local Catholic diocese, and Hubbard's wife Rita. Hubbard flew to his base on Dayman Island to get all the supplies — but by the time he returned, the session had been cancelled. Hubbard was frustrated that his Catholic contacts seemed unconvinced of the science behind psychedelic therapy, while his medical friends remained skeptical of his Catholic associations. Then, a month after the cancelled session, the Montreal psychiatrist reappeared on his doorstep.

"We heard a knock at our door about 8 p.m.," he explained, "and there stood poor dejected Dr. X."

After the session was over, "Dr. X" said "it cost him a great deal of money for his own analysis in becoming a psychiatrist but he considered this of far greater value, in fact, he considers it the greatest development in mental medicine of our day." Hubbard chuckled as he also realized that the poor young doctor was "frightened out of his wits, and even more terrified when he realized that he was facing a priest who could appreciate that his attitude towards the church was a mere ritual and not belief or trust."

As with the Montreal psychiatrist, many of the 1957 LSD sessions took the appearance of public relations exercises; among the first recorded patients at Hollywood Hospital were high-ranking members of the academic and ecclesiastical communities, including a university professor and a Catholic priest.

"I was given a picture of Jesus and asked to look at it and think of who he was," the professor later wrote. But suddenly "the picture starts to change a little bit, to come alive, and then I get scared."

While Hubbard was certainly keen to bring a religious dimension into the sessions, he was careful to utilize LSD to help patients explore past traumas.

"The director [Hubbard] handed me a photograph of my mother, at the sight of which I began to weep silently," the professor continued. "I felt like crying for my mother; she seemed sad and frightened in the picture, not loved and secure."

An hour passed. Hubbard handed the professor a mirror.

"It is hard to describe the feeling of revulsion that this produced," the professor noted. "The face I saw was unsymmetrical and ugly [...] Worst of all, I was completely false." Feelings coursed through the professor as he gazed at his reflection. "I couldn't accept what I saw — couldn't even look the image in the eye [...] I began to see the part my father had played in this. He was always too busy to give the family any time [...] it seemed that he rejected me, and as a result I was rejecting myself."

At that moment, Hubbard brought the professor a flower.

"Look at this flower," he said. "What would happen if you became afraid of life?"

"It would wilt," the professor replied.

Hubbard smiled. "It wilted as you said that."

While the professor claimed some deep insights from this session, he recommended to Hubbard that "those whose intellects are highly trained to be critical and analytical" may need higher doses.

Hubbard would take this note under advisement.

Then, in the autumn of 1957, Hollywood Hospital found itself briefly in the public eye. Robert Sommers, the BC Minister of Forestry, had recently disappeared amid allegations of corruption, and the *Vancouver Province* sent rookie journalist Ben Metcalfe to investigate a tip that Sommers was hiding out at the facility. Metcalfe was unable to locate Sommers, but the building left an impression on him.

"Hollywood Hospital at that time was still famous as a drying-out tank for elite dipsomaniacs," he recalled, "and an air of confidentiality draped the house and grounds like a cloak, night and day."

All of that was about to change in a major way.

In a few short months, the world would finally be introduced to the Acid Room.

Part II: Kaleidoscopic Display of Colours

If the doors of perception were cleansed,
everything would appear to man as it is: infinite.

— William Blake, *The Marriage of Heaven and Hell*

Doug Hepburn
May 16, 1962

Once, he had been the strongest man in the world.

Now he was nothing.

Only ten years earlier, he was a world weightlifting champion, the recipient of several gold medals, and the first man in history to bench press 400, then 450, and then 500 pounds. Now he drifted through the streets of Vancouver's Downtown Eastside in tattered, mismatched clothing, his champion physique having dwindled from 305 pounds to just 120. The main reason for his precipitous decline was booze; born with a club foot and crossed eyes, the young Doug Hepburn was forced to endure multiple painful surgeries throughout his childhood, and became a popular target for bullies. His home life was no better; his father, an abusive alcoholic, left when Hepburn was four, and his mother's series of new husbands wanted little to do with him. Forced out of his own home at eighteen, he turned to physical training as an outlet, a way to transform himself from a scared, physically challenged kid into a champion.

It wasn't enough.

Winning the World Weightlifting Championship in 1953 should have been a cause for celebration, an amazing accomplishment for someone in his position. Instead, he turned to the bottle. Hepburn had never been great with money; the night after his champion-ship win, he slept in a $3-per-night flophouse. He tried his hand at professional wrestling, but abhorred the violence. He tried to open a chain of gyms, including one for women on Commercial Drive. They failed. He was forced to move in with friends, his only income coming from a mail-order bodybuilding course he sold.

"I've only known poverty since I left wrestling," he told a reporter. "Theoretically, I own only the clothes on my back, and the spoon I eat with. They have to leave you that much or you can't live."

As his drinking increased, he became a regular fixture at the Clover Hotel in Cloverdale, regularly consuming fifty or more bottles of beer per day.

"That's where I lost my soul," he later said.

By May 1962, when he turned up on the doorstep of Holly-wood Hospital, he had hit rock bottom.

"Finally, I admitted it," he said. "I suddenly realized — you have a problem you don't understand and you need help."

Having heard about the experimental therapy being conducted inside its walls, Hepburn was intrigued by the promise that it could transform an individual's self-image, reportedly accomplishing in an afternoon what traditional therapy couldn't in years.

"I wish to become a man in the fullest sense," he wrote on his admission form, "so that others can respect and feel that I am an asset, not a detriment, to them. To achieve this ideal will without a shred of a doubt, entail a complete and perpetual ceasation [sic] of alcoholic intake. I think people respect me, for myself, and for what I have accomplished ... "

After meeting with clinic psychedelic therapist John Holloway, Hepburn would have had few illusions about the challenge ahead.

"Tomorrow you're going to have to do something that will be harder than winning ten world championships," Holloway told him. "Because you're going to have to overcome the will that made you a world champion — it has been misdirected and now it is working against you. Tomorrow, under LSD, you are going to have to die.... symbolically."

As was standard, Hepburn stayed overnight in the hospital, fasting and responding to a set of questions for the upcoming session. The next day, he was led into a private room and given 250 micrograms of LSD, dissolved in water and served in a crystal chalice. In attendance was J. Ross MacLean and therapist Frank Ogden. As the drug began to take hold, Hepburn noted, he "was going through a dark valley. I was floating. Coasting down...and down...and there were caverns and rocks and skulls and bones."

Hepburn heard a loud clang — a noise he later discovered was the scratch of the needle on the nearby record player. He reached the bottom of the pit and found himself strapped to the ground, naked and lying on his back.

"And from the forest or jungle or something, they kept coming — these demons," he explained. "And they had pitchforks and it was all Technicolor [...] You can only try and describe it in words."

Terrified, Hepburn found himself being devoured alive. The demons that assailed him, the doctors explained, were his fears. And his drinking, he realized, was a way of coping with them — his abusive childhood, the pain of multiple surgeries, and the lack of self-worth his disabilities had engendered. To become the kind of man he wanted to be, Hepburn realized, he would need to stand up to the horde. Despite the horrifying images, he found his courage and stood strong. Robbed of their power, the demons fled.

After six hours, he was taken to a separate room, where he was encouraged to eat, sleep, and write about the experience.

It would transform the rest of his life.

Four years later, when interviewed by a local newspaper, he noted that he hadn't had a single bottle of beer since his session. He began weightlifting again, opened his own line of gyms, and took up singing as a form of self-therapy. By the age of forty-two, he was back in the spotlight — the subject of movies, television shows, and magazine articles. He became a successful business-man, selling weight training equipment, and even began turning a profit to pay down years of back taxes.

"I must be free," he told a reporter. "I can't work for anybody. I have to be the boss. I have to prove to myself that this new Doug Hepburn can make it in the world of business in the same way the old Doug Hepburn [did]."

Reporters fixated on the remarkable transformation; what had he done to turn his life around? Hepburn wasn't shy about the process; in subsequent years, he offered testimonials advocating for psychedelic therapy. He sat in with a patient him-self in 1963, as an observer. In 1964, his cousin also underwent treatment at Hollywood Hospital; he and a smattering of other patients identified Hepburn as their reason for seeking psyche-delic therapy.

"Having seen Doug's results I cannot help but want the same type of results for myself," his cousin wrote in his admission statement. "With the help of this treatment I hope to become the type of person who has confidence within himself and does not continue to use a false front to cover up insecurity."

By 1993, the sixty-seven-year-old Hepburn was living and working out of a drafty shop along False Creek, in the heart of Vancouver, selling health food and making his own workout equipment, in the company of a black cat named Cupcake. With a bushy moustache and a booming voice, he had managed to rebuild his impressive physique, now weighing in at 237 pounds, and was planning on a weightlifting comeback in the over-sixty-five category. He had also grown more philosophical, becoming a vegetarian and spending periods of time overseas, in India. A screenplay based on his life, called *Magnificent Journey*, was being written. Most of all, Hepburn looked at peace. He had seemingly little need for other people, preferring instead to spend his days and nights in quiet contemplation.

"Fundamentally, I'm a recluse," he told *Province* reporter Tom Hawthorn. "Over in India, they have another name for it. I'm searching for…"

"Privacy?" someone in the shop asked.

"Not privacy," he replied. "Wisdom. But not the wisdom normally recognized in the world. Another kind."

4

MONEY

I went through phases of euphoria and deep sadness as I identified with what seemed like the glory and anguish of all mankind. Life seemed to have a central purpose of love of my fellow man. It was evident that to hurt another person is to hurt ourselves. [...] I sensed that this life is a preparation for something greater which I was experiencing the fringes at.

— Jesse T., Hollywood Hospital patient, fall 1967

DESPITE A RELATIVELY SLOW START in the early part of 1958, business at Hollywood Hospital was picking up.

And when the first patients began to arrive, they found themselves in a hospital ward unlike any they had seen before. By all accounts, the interior was homey, still retaining its turn-of-the-century character. Curiously, the lobby featured a clock that ran backwards — a disconcerting choice for a mental health facility.

Typically, each session started with the administration of Hubbard's carbon dioxide and oxygen (carbogen) mixture, which he believed "tested" the patient's suitability for LSD therapy. Patients would most often arrive the night before, fasting, writing an autobiography outlining their reasons for seeking treatment, and filling out a survey that delved into all manner of personal matters — the deaths of family members, military experience, religion, and sexual and legal history. Patients wrote as much or as little as they wanted, from a few lines to, in one case, an eighty-page document. Some sketched images that helped them express their feelings about themselves. A few wrote poems. Many people struggled to express themselves confidently, choosing words carefully, yet forcefully.

"I never liked my father," one wrote. "I don't think he ever loved me."

"My wife never let me touch her," confessed another.

The next morning, in the presence of Hubbard, MacLean, and a nurse, most received between 300 and 400 micrograms of LSD, served in a crystal chalice (doses ranged from 100 to 1,000 micrograms, depending on the patient). Some had mescaline. Some were given both. Thanks in large part to the Acid Room sessions, the facility's reputation was changing. Gone were the stacks of unpaid bills; for approximately $500 (patients were charged on a sliding scale, plus $18 per day for accommodation), people were beginning to line up for the chance to undergo a life-changing experience. And when they did so, it was in a comfortable room, surrounded by art, music, and empathetic observers who could help guide them through an experience that gave them insight into the root of their addictions or personal conflicts and traumatic pasts. Afterward, they would be taken to a nearby room to decompress, with a nurse checking in every fifteen or thirty minutes. They were given pencil and paper and, if needed, sedatives to counteract the insomnia that often accompanied psychedelics. Patients were required to stay in the hospital for a few days after the experience as they underwent a period of "integration," with therapists helping them reconcile the experience with their lived reality. Follow-ups and a support group were also on offer. A single session seemingly had the potential to supersede years of traditional therapy — and what's more, the changes appeared to stick; in their work with alcoholics MacLean and Hubbard claimed success rates of up to eighty percent.

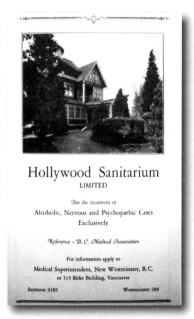

Early advertisement for Hollywood Hospital. Date unknown.

For MacLean, it was a cash cow.

For Al Hubbard, it was the culmination of years of work, a project begun in his humble shed on Dayman Island, that had now expanded into a hospital staffed by professionals, and backed up by a growing body of patient records. And the money started rolling in.

But not everyone was a fan of the new therapeutic techniques.

"Dr MacLean had been under constant pressure from the BC college [of Physicians and Surgeons]," journalist Ben Metcalfe later recalled, "led in no small way by Dr James Tyhurst, then in charge of psychiatry at Vancouver General Hospital, and had several times been called to account for his startling new approach to the art and science of the profession."

Born into a wealthy family, Tyhurst had been an assistant resident at Allan Memorial Institute in Montreal. Perceived as a tyrant by many of his contemporaries (he even insisted on choosing the paint colours on the walls of the UBC psychiatric hospital), Tyhurst became the first head of psychiatry at UBC in 1957. Bald, intimidating, with a square jaw and a pronounced pout, Tyhurst had a murky personal history when it came to psychedelics; he was one of a handful of Canadian academics present at a civil defence forum held at the Waldorf Astoria in Montreal during the summer of 1951 — a forum attended by Canadian military personnel and at least two members of the CIA.

The summit was an attempt by American intelligence to conduct highly covert, and highly unethical research on mind control under the shield of academia — including experiments with sensory deprivation and LSD. Whether Tyhurst himself participated is unclear, but many of his psychiatric contemporaries did, including the University of Montreal's Ewen Cameron. Cameron's experiments proved so extreme that he would later be censured by the scientific community for administering LSD to unwitting, institutionalized participants — many of whom consequently endured years of psychological trauma. In public addresses, Tyhurst often downplayed the usefulness of psychopharmaceuticals (he once told an audience that patients with anxiety should forgo sedative treatment in favour of a few stiff drinks), and when it came to psychedelic therapy, he was openly hostile, having submitted a number of critical briefs to the provincial department of health.

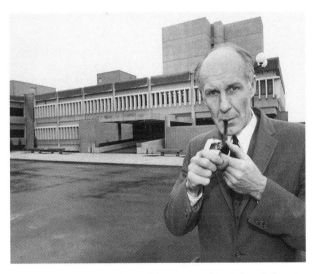

Dr. James Tyhurst in front of the UBC psychiatric hospital, 1968. Image courtesy of the UBC Archives.

At the same time, tensions were growing between Hubbard and his collaborators; the unease surrounding his purchased diploma had intensified, owing to something that Hubbard considered a key feature of Hollywood Hospital's LSD sessions: religion. As a devout Roman Catholic, Hubbard wanted to stimulate spiritual connections, incorporating religious iconography, art, and musical selections that were meant to trigger them. Under Hubbard's influence, subjects described experiences that were spiritual or religious, such as hearing church bells, seeing themselves bathed in a light, or hearing the voice of God. Some of the early experiments with sound even presented passages of the Bible in spoken and musical forms — the most common being a vinyl record of an actor speaking the text of St. Paul's Letters to the Corinthians.

It didn't always work.

One patient of Hubbard's, a Jesuit priest, found himself feeling annoyed rather than entranced.

"It ... sounded ... false, phony," he later complained. "Neither this nor the gospel speaks to me. [...] I want it to mean something — I can make it sound meaningful to everybody but me. [...] This seems to belong to old-time religion, which cannot be my way to God now."

Many of Hubbard's contemporaries, particularly Osmond and Huxley, were also uncomfortable with the overtly religious nature of his sessions, worrying privately that it could undermine patient progress.

"And finally what about Al?" Huxley wrote to Osmond early in 1958. "When you last wrote to me about him, you seemed to think he was a liability rather than an asset, and that it would be a good thing to dissolve the Commission if only to free the more serious researchers from the embarrassment of his carryings on. [...] A week or two ago, Al sent a report on an attempted anti-alcoholism project to be set up under [Catholic Church] auspices, together with notes on a session with [a Catholic] psychiatrist, who had reluctantly submitted to taking LSD-25. Both of them seemed to me to be distressingly absurd, and the report on the session with the psychiatrist was uninhibitedly sectarian."

Though neither worked directly within Hollywood Hospital, both men had begun to feel as if Hubbard had outlived his usefulness within the psychedelic movement. His lack of professional conduct didn't endear their work to academic circles, and his insistence on using LSD to perpetuate Catholic dogma didn't sit well in either secular or religious ones.

"Would it not be best to let Al go his way within the Church?" Huxley continued. "It is evidently there that he feels increasingly at home. It is evident, too, that his loyalty to the Church makes him increasingly anxious to use LSD-25 as an instrument for validating Catholic doctrines and for giving new life to Catholic symbols. Of such, perhaps, is the Kingdom of Heaven — but of such is not the kingdom of Scientific Research."

Hubbard also found himself in conflict with several of Hollywood Hospital's legitimate psychiatrists, including Dr. N. L. Mason Browne, who objected to the religious aspects of Hubbard's sessions. Hubbard himself acknowledged his limitations, openly musing about his waning interest in the sessions — and his own role as scientific director.

"I am completely in accord with you on Dr. Blewett being scientific director and handling communication necessary," he wrote to Hoffer. "I would very much like him to continue to be scientific director as I am afraid, and have been for some time, that my regard for science, as an end within itself, is diminishing as time goes on."

But it wasn't just devotion to Catholic pieties that drove him; what now occupied much of Hubbard's focus was the pursuit of money. Hollywood Hospital was turning a decent profit, but for Hubbard, it wasn't enough. He wanted to go bigger, musing in his letters about establishing a network of psychedelic clinics up and down the West Coast. To that end, he began criss-crossing the continent once again, pursuing investments from a "number of large corporations," and trying to chase down funding from the Rock-efeller family.

In Saskatchewan, many of the up-and-coming pioneers of psychedelic psychiatry were undergoing their first official experiences, including Canadians Duncan Blewett and Nick Chwelos. At Hollywood, these early sessions focused largely on alcoholics; Brian Paterson, a candy salesman who had been in and out of the facility for years due to problem drinking, used his session to confront deep-rooted family trauma. Brendan Riggs, a stockbroker, entered the Acid Room hoping to curb his excessive drinking, and instead left amid a full-blown crisis of conscience over the predatory nature of his work. Although treating alcoholics was the hospital's mandate, some early Hollywood patients had no connection to alcoholism at all; one, Amanda Williamson, underwent treatment because it would "help me think clearer." Another, Corey Baker, an ABC News reporter from New York, went in hoping it would fix his marriage. Under MacLean's guidance, both he and his wife Emily underwent a simultaneous LSD trip, where they confronted years of resentment, a non-existent sex life, and his multiple infidelities.

"We are still cooking with d-Lysergic acid diethylamide at our house," Baker wrote in a letter, "the strains that threatened to blow us apart individually and collectively have all but disappeared. Each new day (and each day looks new) has brought us closer to-gether [sic] in renewal. I credit your skillful guidance for the whole new world we have discovered."

Judging from several follow-up letters, the couple's new outlook seems to have been a long-lasting one.

"Everybody has been remarking on how well [Emily] looks," he continued, "and indeed she is blooming. For the first time too she is able to talk of many things that would have been taboo before. I hadn't realized that such a dramatic change was possible."

During this period, the musical selections used in each session became more standardized. Ranging in style from classical to folk, the records were typically those capable of eliciting an emotional response — anger, joy, sadness, or nostalgia. Typically, a nurse (or, in some cases, Hubbard's wife Rita) would choose from an approved list, including Mahler's First Symphony, *Songs of the South*, and Ravel's *Pavane for a Dead Princess*. And as 1958 turned into 1959, the slow dribble of patients requesting LSD therapy turned into a deluge. Hollywood Hospital was entering its boom years. In early January, the facility hired more staff and held a series of monthly seminars to familiarize them with MacLean and Hubbard's evolving treatment approach. Al Hubbard gave a presentation on the history of psychedelic compounds. Dr. D.C. MacDonald outlined the success and methodology of psychedelic treatment in facilities across Canada. Another psychiatrist, R.L. Swarovski, detailed the intricacies of a nurse's duties before, during, and after a session. And at the core of those seminars was a clear message: Hollywood Hospital was entering a new era — one that would embrace innovative, and sometimes unorthodox, methods.

"We must never be content with our 'status quo,'" MacLean told his staff, "but must constantly seek a better way [...] No organization is able to stand still in the face of changing times and conditions. It will either go forward or backward and without timely changes the only course will be a backward one."

"I enjoy the work very much, and it probably should have been carried out this way long ago," Hubbard remarked with satisfaction, "but in those days we did not have such a fine group of doctors as we have here to work with."

His vision, it seemed, had taken hold.

Unfortunately, Al Hubbard's days at Hollywood Hospital were numbered.

Angela Sucher
Sept 26, 1964

That summer, for a few, intoxicating days, Angela Sucher had felt like a woman.

Not a mother. Not a companion. Not some grotesque biological receptacle for a husband she didn't love, and at whose touch she regularly recoiled.

"I was beautiful and cared for my body as I never had before," she later wrote. "I was kind and loving especially to my husband who knew of everything, I had energy even for the lowest tasks in the household. I became feminine in the way my father had always wanted me to be, playing little games and enjoying them instead of considering them an indignity to my human integrity. I submitted and wanted nothing else but to submit."

She was a thirty-two-year-old mother of four, recently enrolled at Simon Fraser University, eager to lift herself out of a monotonous home life, with the goal of someday getting a Master's degree in linguistics. He was her professor, a man of letters she had just met, and greatly respected — until that respect blossomed into something else.

"In many ways it seemed like my love for him brought out all of my potential," she continued.

Though their association was brief, it was unlike anything Angela had ever experienced, filling a deep need that had been unmet for decades. Though she was ambitious, independent, and highly intelligent, pursuing higher education when only nine percent of Canada's female population was enrolled at university, a preoccupation with conventional notions of womanhood had dominated Angela's thoughts since childhood. Born in prewar Berlin, she grew up in the shadow of the emerging Nazi party, and of a tyrannical father who regularly brutalized his wife and children.

"My parents had almost indoctrinated me from my earliest childhood with the idea that I was the clumsiest creature under the sun," she wrote. "So any physical activity became torture to me. [...] I was too clumsy, not wellgrowned enough, too much of a shrew, not at all charmingly feminine because when I wanted something I asked for it instead of choosing a flattering way around the question." She would, according to her father, "never find a husband and if I did, God help him."

Often, his abuse would turn physical, and Angela found herself deliberately provoking her father, to spare her mother and brother.

"On these occasions I never uttered a murmur," she noted. "I would have rather bitten my tongue than give him that satisfaction."

Like all German children, she was required to join the Hitler Youth, marching in uniform and singing patriotic songs like "Sacred Fatherland." By night, she and her family huddled in the cellar as Allied bombs fell. Despite continuing academic excellence, and participation in all manner of extracurricular activities, her insecurities began manifesting at school, where they were seized upon by her peers; at a year-end dance, a group of students scrawled a verse next to her photo in their annual commemorative magazine:

> *Oh how I am angry,*
> *Oh how I could cry,*
> *Everybody has a man,*
> *Everyone but I.*

"It was quite true," she admitted, "and might have been a good motto for my whole life."

Despite her lamentations, she did prove popular with men; after some experience "necking" in her teens, she fell hopelessly in love with a Catholic priest at the age of seventeen. Then she received a scholarship to a school in the US, and it expanded her romantic horizons.

"I think this year was the only one during which I was carelessly young," she explained.

"I had for the first time the idea that I was a girl. For some reason the American boys seemed to like European girls and were also prepared to spoil them in sharp contrast to their European counterparts."

At twenty, she fell in love with an American medical student. Their early sexual encounters were, by her own admission "pleasant but as far as I was concerned very unsuccessful". After that, she returned to Berlin, and sought out the attention of a much older man — thirty-nine to her twenty-two — in hopes of increasing her own level of sexual experience.

"It was just as unsuccessful," she explained, "although this man was determined to 'awaken' me as he put it. I became quite annoyed with his determination."

As she explored new connections, her desire for them only increased — as did her insecurities. She soon found herself unable to look in the mirror, focusing on a series of perceived flaws in her body and personality. The same preoccupation with femininity remained, and began to feed upon itself.

"When I look in the mirror, which I hardly ever do, I find so many faults that I am hesitant to show myself in a bathing suit in front of a bunch of people," she wrote.

Nonetheless, she soon found herself being pursued by a young man from a good family, a young man with an even temperament and a seemingly promising future, managing one of Germany's largest dairies — someone who, in her words, was "good-looking in an unglamorous way." Although he had initially expressed interest in one of her friends, the pair kept up a correspondence for several years, and little by little, his attention began to seem like something more. But for her, "there was no romantic element to the correspondence."

The quest for a robust intellectual and romantic connection had dominated Angela's thoughts throughout her twenties, but so far had resulted in nothing but a string of disappointing suitors. And by that point, she began to fear that the problem lay with her: that she was too demanding, that she was too picky, that she was "sexually frigid," that she was too clumsy and too direct to conform to society's ideals of womanhood. The words of her father, her mother, her classmates were all pointing to a clear course of action: take what you can get.

So, when the young dairy manager eventually made his romantic interests clear, that's what she did.

"After he left I contemplated the situation and came to the conclusion that he would make a very good husband," she explained. "So everything seemed perfect, and I decided not to wait for love and be sorry ten years later — especially since my chances were not very good anyway."

The marriage was bloodless; although her husband is referenced dozens of times in Angela's patient files, his name is never mentioned. The couple moved to Canada shortly afterward, but once they were settled, their home life quickly grew monotonous. Outside Germany, her husband's prospects were lean, and the ambition he had once shown evaporated. Eking out a meagre existence in a Vancouver rooming house, Angela began to regret ever leaving home.

"I had been told so often that I would make my future husband henpecked," she reflected, "that I agreed to everything for many years against my better judgment. Out of this fear."

Angela gave birth to four children, but her sexual involvement with her husband — never particularly enjoyable, even before parenthood — became unbearable.

"Our relationship for ten years may best be described as mutual masturbation followed by a quick deposit of matter where it belongs," she remarked bitterly. "This proven method brings me a localized sensation and physical satisfaction and makes me shudder when it is all over. I submit to it because it is my marital duty or because it is the only kind of sex available to me, the only kind I am capable of. [...] Sometimes every inch of my skin longs for something that never comes."

In the summer of 1964, that "something" arrived, in the form of her professor on the campus at SFU. For the first time, she was engaging with someone who was her intellectual equal, and she was bewitched by the experience.

"I seemed to be drowning in my own feelings," she noted, "and was incapable of controlling it only in the slightest way."

Unable to keep these feelings to herself, Angela confessed the attraction to her professor. He didn't feel the same.

"And I saw very soon that my idol had clay feet," she wrote. "He was only a year older than I am and in many ways not as mature, uncompromising and strictly honest as I wanted him to be. I came to the conclusion that nobody could ever be what I expected my ideal to be and realized for the first time that I had been trying to find God in men."

It was an insight that proved transformational, and in time her feelings toward her professor changed into something warmer and more expansive.

"This insight cured me of my misconceptions that I had dragged around with me all my life and I was grateful to this man for not having been able to give me the illusion I was expecting," she wrote. "And out of this gratefulness grew a new feeling for him that I can only identify as true love, namely the complete acceptance of a person on his terms with everything he is and is not. It did not matter anymore that he was different than my ideals, it was enough that he was himself."

It's difficult to say, given her language, whether the affair was physical or simply emotional, but in any event, it came to a swift end. And as the months went on, Angela found herself slipping back into her old life, her old habits, and her old feelings. In the wake of her loss, she closed herself off even more than before. She wondered repeatedly if she was a failure as a woman, and lamented her inability to love her husband the way she had briefly loved the professor. There was a woman locked inside her, Angela wrote — behind all the insecurities, all the guilt, all the childhood suffering.

"I was always vaguely aware of her," she said, "but now I am certain she was on parole for a few days in the summer and she finds it terribly hard to have to go back into her prison for no reason."

When Angela arrived at Hollywood Hospital in September 1964, on the advice of her husband, it was, according to her admission form, so that "I can actually be helped to overcome a problem of sexual frigidity."

"Clinically she is of high average to superior I.Q.," noted the doctor, D. C. MacDonald. "She is ambitious, and no doubt will tend to 'intellectualize' to excess in a psychedelic treatment experience. […] She does not appear neurotic, but I believe she would need a fairly large dose of drug material, 700–800 mmg, to reduce her defenses."

On the morning of Sept 26, Angela Sucher was led into one of the psychedelic treatment rooms at Hollywood Hospital, and given 900 milligrams of mescaline in the company of Frank Ogden and Ross MacLean. Clutched in her hands were photos of her parents, and several records she hoped to hear. As was standard, she was given a blanket and fitted with an eye mask.

As was often the case with patients, the mescaline didn't agree with her. After her stomach calmed, a record was placed on the stereo; it was Mahler's First Symphony, but to Angela, it sounded like "Sacred Fatherland," the Nazi anthem she had been forced to sing as a child. Suddenly, it all came rushing back: the Hitler Youth emblem, the war, the nights huddled in her basement as the Allied bombs fell.

"I hated Hitler for trying to destroy the hearts of children," she later wrote. "I was trained to be heroic and put on a uniform. I hated that uniform and I knew that I was a child trampled under the crowd of the adults playing war. Without any consideration for the children. I was full of hate for the whole regime."

They changed the music shortly afterward, to a folk song, and Angela's thoughts turned wistful. In her mind, she could see the professor off in the distance. She ran toward him, feeling playful, and when he turned, she stepped back, giggling.

"You didn't catch me again," she laughed. After a moment, she added, "I always catch myself."

As the music changed to Ravel's "Bolero," she began to squirm in discomfort, pounding the couch with her fists.

"What I need now is a knight in shining armor," she said finally. On the horizon, where the professor had once stood, she saw just such a knight. But when she approached and lifted the visor, the face that peered back from within was her own.

As the experience drew to a close, Angela spent several hours alone in her room, reflecting on notions of womanhood, society, sexuality, and self-worth.

"Intellectuality has been the only mode of living in which I have been successful," she wrote. "I will have to force myself back into it to rescue a measure of self-respect. If I can't be a woman I will just have to make the best of trying to be a human being. I am sorry to sound so disappointed, but I am blaming nobody but myself for this failure."

Her despair was short-lived.

By the following morning, she was in high spirits. And, over the following year, during a series of follow-up appointments, she came to regard the session as one of the most important moments of her life. As far as she was concerned, her session in the Acid Room had been a victory; she had realized the importance of intellectual connection, and recognized the value of her own intelligence.

"How wonderful it is," she wrote, "to know oneself!"

Her feelings about her husband remained unchanged — by her final letter in 1965, she was relieved that he would be away in Germany for three weeks. And though she had come to acknowledge that her unfulfilling marriage was a large part of the problem, a commitment to her children kept her from leaving.

But it appears she did find a solution to the "sexual frigidity" noted on her intake form; during a follow-up appointment in the spring of 1964, she sexually propositioned her therapist.

Several months later, she did it again.

5

ANY COLOUR YOU LIKE

The only word I can use to describe the experience, Beautiful! Beautiful! To be taken to the depths of despair, degradation & then to be lifted to the heights […] Life & Death loose [sic] their fear. Each a separate entity & yet all in One [sic]. In the early hours of the morning following LSD I saw the galaxy of stars, their beauty unsurpassed, eyes open or shut. Never before revealed to me like then.

— Jeremy K., Hollywood Hospital patient, summer 1970

IN THE OPENING MONTHS OF 1959, LSD therapy continued to explode.

During this period, Hollywood Hospital handled two dozen cases, with more patients streaming in every month. By now, Ross

MacLean was involved in more than twenty different businesses —
some affiliated with the hospital, some not — using his increased
means to purchase a ranch in Ashcroft, BC, and move his family
(now four children strong) into Casa Mia, the iconic Vancouver
mansion once owned by millionaire bootlegger Henry Reifel. He
drove a brand-new Cadillac, while the flamboyant Hubbard purchased a two-toned Rolls-Royce. Psychedelic psychiatry became so
popular that a handful of celebrities and musicians from south of the
border (including Andy Williams and Guy Mitchell) also snuck up
to take part — though, for the sake of discretion, they stayed at Casa
Mia with the MacLean family.

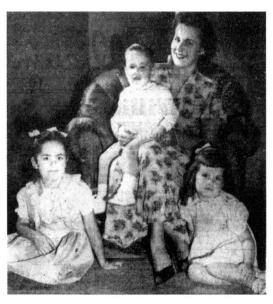

The MacLean family, 1951.

However, despite its success, Hollywood Hospital had a public relations problem.

James Tyhurst and the BC College of Physicians had ramped up their attacks, and consequently provincial health minister Bert Price was privately threatening to withdraw Hollywood's bed subsidy. Desperate, Ross MacLean hired William Clancy and Associates, a high-end publicity firm considered the resident experts on currying government favour. Clancy tasked senior associate Clare Anderson, a former *Province* journalist, with improving Hollywood's image in the public eye, and Anderson in turn went in search of a local reporter who would be willing to portray the hospital in as favourable a light as possible.

He found Ben Metcalfe.

The forty-year-old journalist hadn't set foot in Hollywood Hospital since staking it out on the trail of the disgraced forestry minister back in 1957, but Anderson's offer intrigued him.

"You've been almost everywhere in this world," Anderson grinned. "Now how would you like to go out of this world for a spell?"

It was more than the adventurous Metcalfe could resist. In the summer of 1959, he met with MacLean and Hubbard, to get a sense of the operation and talk strategy. They settled on a six-part series, to be published in the *Province* in early September that would showcase the hospital's unique treatment approach, with Metcalfe sitting in on patient sessions and reporting their results. But Metcalfe wasn't content to simply be an observer. He went to editor William Forst and told him that he needed to undergo LSD therapy himself.

"They were not so much skeptical as they were bewildered," he later said, "but they agreed to let me go ahead if I would sign a waiver releasing the *Province* from any responsibility for my fate, which I in turn agreed to do."

Metcalfe never signed the release. But, in August of 1959, he arrived at Hollywood Hospital to check himself in. Over several days, he observed a handful of patient sessions — an alcoholic mother, an anxiety sufferer, a young man so afflicted with depression that he could barely walk. And then it was time for him to undergo a session of his own.

In the presence of Hubbard, MacLean, and nurse Leona Kirby, he sipped 400 micrograms of LSD from a crystal chalice and lay back on the couch. The drug took effect within fifteen minutes, and suddenly Metcalfe found himself captivated by his hands.

"What wonderful things the hands are," he said.

Then he burst into tears, crying into a pillow for more than five minutes.

"This is all repressed material coming up," Hubbard said gently. "This is what we bury to become men."

"Great waves of meaning carried me away," Metcalfe later wrote. "I saw this earthly reality falling away from me in descending spirals, my wife, my children, my friends, the city, all parting from my memory of them like flakes of multicoloured snow vanishing in darkness while I sped upward."

Covering his eyes, he roamed through history with Shakespeare and Cervantes, the music played by Nurse Kirby bringing him to extremes of emotion and manifesting itself in every colour of the rainbow.

"Words are not enough for this!" he shouted.

His own experience lasted eight hours, after which he was taken to a recovery room to write and decompress, "watching whole gardens of blossoms grow out of the curtains, papering the walls with strange maps and studying the antics of impossible creatures romping along the wainscotting."

The following day, he observed one final session. This time, it was a married couple — a white psychiatrist dubbed "Dr. Stan", and his South Asian wife, named Positari. Although they had come to partake of "the Experience" out of professional curiosity, it was clear to

Metcalfe from the outset that their marriage was in trouble. They drank from the chalice, and after approximately fifteen minutes, she began weeping softly. Dr. Stan got up from the couch, knelt in front of her, and said, "It's okay, honey."

"It was their last real contact for four hours," Metcalfe wrote. "What happened in between was a poignant drama of two individuals, bound to each other by law and a few emotions beforehand, but drifting through the heavens and hells of their own minds quite apart."

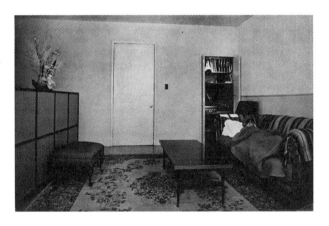

The interior of the Acid Room, circa 1965.

As Positari wept, her husband thrashed on the couch, shouting about truth and lies, and attempting to get a handle on his senses.

"I felt sorry for him," she said, to nobody in particular.

This scene continued for a further four hours, the couple sequestered in their own private worlds, bouncing between sadness and elation.

Then, suddenly, Dr. Stan called out, "Darling!"

She got to her feet and embraced him, laying her head on his shoulder.

After a moment, she asked: "Do you still want to beat me?"

"No," he said, through tears. "I would never do that. I want to come back. Back to you."

"The scene was intimate but not embarrassing least of all to them," Metcalfe wrote. "The emotion of it filled the room."

As planned, Metcalfe's series appeared in the pages of the *Province* in early September, and, in his words, the articles "turned the town on its ear."

Hollywood Hospital enrolments went up even more sharply. The paper was flooded with letters to the editor — both critical and supportive. In the meantime, Tyhurst and the BC College of Physicians vowed to draft their own report.

"It is true that there is no final theory why LSD works as it does," Ross MacLean argued in the *Province*. "So far, we can only go by results, and so far the results are exceptional, both here and at Saskatoon, the centre of world research into LSD."

But it wasn't just Hollywood Hospital that had made the papers; stories about psychedelic therapy were everywhere. In a 1959 issue of *Look* magazine, actor Cary Grant was candid about undergoing more than a hundred LSD sessions, crediting it with saving his health and his marriage. Crooner Andy Williams was similarly effusive in his praise. Then Canadian researchers Duncan Blewett and Nick Chwelos published the *Handbook for the Therapeutic Use of LSD-25*. The book was — and remains — the authoritative guide to psychedelic psychiatry, laying out in intimate detail the inner workings of the Acid Room, and in its opening pages, it singles out the work of one Al Hubbard.

"It will be obvious to the careful reader," says the foreword, "but it is a pleasure to acknowledge here as well, the debt which the authors owe to the work of Dr. A. M. Hubbard and the help of Dr. H. Osmond."

"Most people are walking in their sleep," Hubbard said in an interview. "Turn them around, start them in the opposite direction and they wouldn't even know the difference. But give them a good dose of LSD and let them see themselves for what they are."

Naturally, there was a backlash. In the wake of the controversy surrounding Metcalfe's articles, which were picked up in papers across Canada, the federal government and Sandoz itself decided to take a second look at the distribution of their supplies. Hubbard and Tyhurst locked horns publicly in late 1959 — though it seems Hubbard managed to hold his own.

"Al Hubbard did not come out of his wrangle with the Professor of Psychiatry in Vancouver too badly," Osmond noted in a letter to Aldous Huxley. "Indeed he did very well considering how formidable his opponent is known to be. As I feared, his correspondence course PhD was not wholly approved of, although undoubtedly legal. Al was nonplussed by this. It had not struck him that regarding a scientific qualification recognition by peers might be most important. However he hasn't come to much harm."

With public scrutiny increasing, many of psychedelic therapy's pioneers became increasingly worried about the future of their work. For years, a schism had been developing between serious academics like Osmond and MacLean, and dreamers like Hubbard. MacLean knew that Hollywood Hospital needed more than just good PR; they needed scientific legitimacy, and that without it, the antics of men like Hubbard could undermine the movement as a whole.

"I only hope that some of our newer developments will make it less profitable for the incompetent and crooked," Osmond wrote in another letter to Huxley. "Many psychiatrists are either unsuited or insufficiently trained for the work. The trouble is that the demand is considerable and the less able or more unscrupulous can make much money. Medicine has a long and depressing history of substandard professional work about which we have been incredibly slow about doing very much."

While MacLean prepared patient data for publication, Al Hubbard's mind was wandering far beyond the walls of Hollywood Hospital. A number of sources place Hubbard's departure sometime in 1959, but in fact he continued working with patients and corresponding on hospital stationery through 1960 and into 1961. Nonetheless, he was slowly becoming a fringe figure in therapeutic circles; the day-to-day reality of treating patients had grown steadily less interesting, and now, once again, he yearned for something bigger.

Then, in early 1960, a man with dark hair and a moustache walked through the front doors and asked for a job. He had no medical training — in fact, no formal experience at all — though this didn't seem to bother him.

"I told them I was well qualified to work as a guide into 'inner space' because I'd flown flying boats and survived helicopter crashes," he chuckled. "I told them adventure was my game."

Born aboard a passenger train near Toronto, he had worked as a deckhand on banana boats and flown airplanes during the Second World War. Back in 1953, he set an altitude record by taking the impossibly dangerous step of removing much of the fuel from his airplane's engine. He would go on to be friends with science fiction author Arthur C. Clarke, as well as the author of a nationally syndicated newspaper column who took to calling himself "Doctor Tomorrow."

His name was Frank Ogden, and he was about to take Hollywood Hospital in a new direction.

Part III: Most Severe Crisis

The martyrs go hand in hand into the arena; they are crucified alone.

— Aldous Huxley, *The Doors of Perception*

Patrick Sealgair
October 17, 1967

A few months before Patrick Sealgair entered high school, his mother hit him in the face with a hammer.

It was the most recent act of abuse in a pattern that stretched back to his childhood, and this abuse, Patrick noted, is what likely resulted in the "problem" that had brought him to Hollywood Hospital.

"What I hoped to accomplish, through therapy, was an end to my homosexuality," he wrote in his pre-treatment autobiography. "Guilt about my past history and recurring desires for men, during my marriage, had caused me to allow and even to encourage my wife to divorce me, in spite of my love for her."

For Patrick, there was a straight line between this boyhood abuse and the "compulsive" homosexual behaviour that now occupied much of his free time.

"Constant physical beatings at the hands of my mother could have caused my sexual deviation," he continued. "My sexual attitudes are a direct result of puritanical education, at home and in school."

Despite his past, Patrick arrived at the hospital as a thirty-seven-year-old New York actor and playwright with above-average intelligence and a dose of self-esteem big enough that it often tipped into arrogance.

"More often than not, people are shocked to hear that I am 37, nearly 38, taking me for about ten years younger," he bragged. "I do too many things too well [...] cook, keep house, sew, decorate, build, create, blend, dance, act, write, and handle most jobs as well or better than most. I'm a good host and people seem to enjoy being my guest or in my company socially, certainly more for the most part than I enjoy them."

Born into a lower-class Irish family, he had been engaging, compulsively and regularly, in sex acts with men since early adolescence. In the months leading up to his arrival at Hollywood Hospital, he had fallen in love with two different young men — one twenty-two, the other twenty-four. His contact with women had been brief, sporadic, and largely unfulfilling, with the exception of a woman he had married for a period of three years back in his early twenties. In spite of this, Patrick was unwilling to fully accept his sexual orientation, and had come seeking LSD therapy in hopes of affecting a heterosexual conversion.

"To date, I still can't honestly say that I've accepted myself as a homosexual any more than I can honestly state that I've ever been otherwise," he wrote. "Often, I have felt that I am at a strange midpoint between two worlds, never really in either [...] What I would hope to accomplish through LSD is an understanding of the causes of my homosexuality, either ending it or learning a degree of acceptance or participation other than the compulsiveness I now have to live with. I would like to be able to live my life constructively but I've known little freedom from this compulsive behavior, as time goes by I know less."

His childhood in New York was, as described in his autobiography, horrific — abuse at the hands of not just his alcoholic parents, but his older brother, and by the time he was twelve, he had been placed in a Catholic home for boys, where he began exploring his sexuality with other young men.

"The boy was my age and the experience was mastabatory [sic], without orgasim [sic] on my part, in a sort of field lavortory [sic]," he recalled, of his first encounter. "It had been preceeded [sic] by a few vague sex investigation-curiosity type contacts with other playmates, in earlier years, all stimulated by dark isolated places and being alone with one friend. I believe I've always loved my friends too well, invariably desiring sex contact. I think this is largely due to having been affection starved at home."

These explorations continued into high school, where he was, at first, an exceptional student. But when Patrick was transferred to Cathedral College — a seminary — he found his grades slipping substantially.

"I was one of the top students in the class and then I was admitted to Cathedral College and that was for the study of priesthood," he explained, during an interview with his New York psychiatrist. "And for the first six months there, for the first time in my life I failed the subjects, not only one, I failed every goddamn one right down the line."

He never finished high school.

In the years that followed, he managed to liberate himself from his family, moving west to California, where he worked a variety of odd jobs and began pursuing theatre and film.

"As far as physical appearance was concerned, I did not fancy myself as a Hollywood star," he noted. "I had no illusion about being beautiful, so as a result the motion picture industry fascinated me as an industry, I didn't know where I could possibly fit and at that time I didn't think of myself as an actor in the business."

Nonetheless, he landed a series of bit parts in movies and began to explore his first love: playwriting. He was increasingly promiscuous during these years, finding himself popular with men in Los Angeles's underground club scene.

"In the 'gay' world, I've recently been astounded at my success," he later wrote, "being able to attract and 'go home with' just about everyone I wanted."

But these successes just felt empty.

"Next to never, do I find anyone who has anything about them, in the way of ethics or standards, that I can admire," he admitted. "Being physically attractive for them is so artificial and so dependent on a wide variety of personal phantasizing [sic]. I know how to succeed sexually but find myself feeling increasingly emptier afterwards."

During this period, he ran into trouble with the law on two different occasions; the first, after calling his landlady an "old bitch" following a dispute over unpaid rent, and the second after he was lured into a compromising position by a member of the Los Angeles vice squad. In both cases, the charges were dropped, and Patrick ultimately returned to New York City in hopes of pursuing a career as a playwright. Never more than a few steps from poverty, he took jobs with a market research company to keep the lights on, developing a series of short plays based on his life and experiences. During this period, he also attempted to distance himself from his promiscuous past, attending psychotherapy and attempting to cultivate connections with women. Then, at the age of twenty-four, he met a woman while dancing at a New York nightspot. It was, he claimed, "love at first sight," and ten days later, they were married — over the strenuous objections of her mother.

It was the only heterosexual relationship Patrick ever attempted.

Unsurprisingly, it didn't last. On multiple occasions, he later claimed that those married years were the best of his life. But in reality their sex life was sporadic and unfulfilling, and his wife, already dealing with a serious anxiety disorder, couldn't cope with the stress of her husband's wandering eye. After three-and-a-half years, they separated.

Feeling empty and confused, Patrick quickly returned to cruising, frequenting Manhattan's gay bars and again finding consistent success — though these encounters often left him even emptier than before.

"However, that is not really what I wanted at any time, always looking for that one person," he wrote. "In this I fail miserably. Those I select as 'the one person' usually like and respect me, while going off with someone else. Apparently, I lack emotional appeal. Perhaps, I present too much of a challenge in being good at too damm [sic] many things, it's hard for people to be 'one up' on me. I've mellowed with the years," he admitted in a moment of self-realization, "but I'm still too outspoken and opinionated."

This outspoken attitude also occasionally got him into trouble at work; recently, he had been fired from a market research job for "exploding at a fool of a supervisor."

Though Patrick himself had been treated respectfully and held up as a model employee to the others, "[i]t was sickening to see them let him get away with walking on them and when he [the supervisor] made the mistake of speking [sic] to me in an uncivil fashion, I promptly read him out, loud and clear, in front of the entire office and in no uncertain terms."

His boyhood experiences had birthed a bold streak and a lifelong inability to abide bullying, and since his teenage years, he had never been one to shy away from a fight; the night before he arrived at Hollywood Hospital, he ended up in a tussle with the jilted ex-partner of his twenty-four-year-old lover.

"The only thing I fear is quite real, that of being arrested as a homosexual in patronizing 'gay' bars," he noted. "In fact I had a nightmare, just last night, in which I came out of a bar where I thought I was avoiding a possible 'raid', only to find myself faced with a gun and then pointed out to be one of those to be arrested because I was wearing a leather jacket. The terror was so real that I woke up."

His fears were well founded.

The *Diagnostic and Statistical Manual of Mental Disorders*, released in 1952 and considered the authoritative guide to mental health, classified homosexuality as a psychiatric disorder, listed alongside conditions like fetishism and pedophilia. In Canada and the United States, homosexuality was also a criminal offence, one which could be used as pretext to be denied entry into the country, to be arrested, or to be fired from one's job. That Patrick sought LSD therapy in hopes of conversion wasn't unusual; since 1960, a handful of gay patients had come to Hollywood Hospital — some for conversion, others for perspective.

In October 1967, he stepped into the Acid Room. On account of his superior intelligence, he was given a whopping 300 micrograms of LSD and 400 micrograms of mescaline, and made to lie down on the couch with his eyes covered.

The first sensation he experienced was nausea — a common response. It continued intermittently through the first four hours of his session, leading him to thrash on the couch in agony.

"To describe the 'experience' is to describe the phantasy of my life," he later wrote. "All of the horrors I made up were turned into colors, shapes and textures, some of the meanings of which I must honestly say I don't yet understand. [...] I remember laughing and thrilling to the sound of music and the array of colors, just as I have in my life."

"Can't have it both ways," he murmured, laying on the couch in the Acid Room, "has to be one way or the other. Which way, though?"

He nodded his head and began to sob. By now, the nausea had become overwhelming, and he moaned, "Oh my god what pain that is." Then, in a momentary loss of control, he urinated on himself.

"I know what caused the nausea," he wrote, "self loathing and/or lack of love, inside myself or myself and consequently for all men and women. Consequently, with and as part of this nausea there were gas pains in my stomach. [...] The gas was the cloud I continued up in my search for love."

Shouting, he got to his feet, removing his soiled pyjamas and standing naked in the centre of the room.

"Look at this fantasy mess!" he declared. "Got to get up & let the fresh air through it."

But he could see through the pain and nausea, see the pain of his upbringing, the pain stemming from his own lack of self-acceptance. Fortunately, it subsided by halfway through the session, and Patrick was able to settle, his thoughts focusing on his parents, his upbringing, his future, himself. The next morning, he awoke feeling, in his words, "newborn."

"I had never accepted the 'gas', in the homosexual, in my life as being a real part of me," he wrote afterward, "could not do so in delerium [sic]. I wanted to be normal and had to get back to that reality. It all makes such sense now."

"It wasn't sinful," he added, of his sexuality, "only in my mother's eyes, and I reinforced it to show my love for my mother."

His correspondence with Hollywood Hospital following the session was brief, but in it, he spoke of wanting to help other gay men in his life — his twenty-four-year-old lover and several of their friends — achieve some measure of perspective.

"Why will I go on?" he wrote. "So that I may help others find themselves because it is only in loving others that you love your-self, but first I had to learn to love myself again to become one part again."

It is unknown if Patrick Sealgair succeeded in this goal. It is impossible to say if he achieved any measure of success as a New York playwright. But one thing is for certain — he entered the Acid Room seeking conversion, and instead he emerged with some-thing much more valuable: insight.

When J. Ross MacLean published his first paper on the use of LSD and mescaline at Hollywood Hospital in 1965, he took a moment to note the results with gay patients.

"Few homosexuals in our group have attained a satisfactory heterosexual adjustment," he explained, "yet many have derived marked benefit in terms of insight, acceptance of role, reduction of guilt and associated psychosexual liabilities."

Homosexuality wasn't officially removed from the *DSM* until 1980.

6

US AND THEM

When one has been through an LSD Experience — you are a changed person — and you will never be the same again […] However I know the battle remains largely to be fought — my conscious self is back in control and the imprinting of 45 years of life is going to be extremely difficult to modify and change and yet I only hope and have confidence that I have been shown the way and can make progress towards changing myself back into the human being that I was meant to be.

— Justina D., Hollywood Hospital patient, summer 1959

IT WAS EARLY 1962, and Al Hubbard was about to make the biggest mistake of his life: driving his Rolls-Royce through downtown Boston, he decided to stop at the home of a young Harvard psychology professor named Timothy Leary. Hubbard had gotten word that Leary and his colleague Richard Alpert were conducting experiments involving psilocybin mushrooms, and, sensing a kindred spirit, decided to make an introduction.

"He blew in laying down the most incredible atmosphere of mystery and flamboyance, and really impressive bullshit," Leary recalled. "He was pissed off. His Rolls Royce had broken down on the freeway, so he went to a pay phone and called the company in London. That's what kind of guy he was. He started name-dropping like you wouldn't believe … claimed he was friends with the Pope."

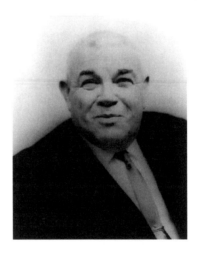

Al Hubbard, circa 1960s.

The Captain wanted mushrooms, and, producing a briefcase filled with LSD, he asked if Leary might be willing to trade. When

Leary agreed, Hubbard pulled the ever-present tank of carbogen from his trunk and encouraged Leary to give it a try. Leary immediately took Hubbard at his word and decided that he would begin incorporating LSD into his own experiments.

"The thing that impressed me," Leary said, "is on one hand he looked like a carpetbagger con man, and on the other he had these most-impressive people in the world on his lap, basically backing him."

In the year since taking his leave from Hollywood Hospital, Hubbard had been busy. His dream of creating a chain of psychedelic research centres was still firmly in his mind, and, in March, he advised Osmond that a network would soon be springing up all over the West Coast.

And, he added, he wanted Osmond and Hoffer to advise.

Osmond (who had since left Saskatchewan for Princeton) wasn't enthusiastic.

"While we are always keen to encourage the active and enterprising," Osmond wrote to Aldous Huxley, "we don't want to put our names on note paper headings again until someone is actually doing something in an organised way. Al has an admirable gift of optimism and enthusiasm essential for any enterprise, but one may have some difficulty in distinguishing his honest hopes from what others really intend to do."

In addition, Hubbard and his friend Myron Stolaroff joined forces to establish the International Foundation for Advanced Study (IFAS) in Menlo Park, California. Stolaroff, a Silicon Valley pioneer, in turn invited other technical wizards to take part, including Doug Englebart, inventor of, among other things, the computer mouse. The IFAS followed the same basic guidelines as Hollywood Hospital — the same methods Hubbard had employed in the Acid Rooms of New Westminster were used to treat American patients: the carbogen, the questionnaire, the therapists, and the LSD. There are rumours he brought celebrities and business moguls to the facility, or to his house on Dayman Island. At one time, he reportedly had 10,000 doses of Sandoz LSD in a storage locker in Zurich, until the Swiss government found out he wasn't paying duty and deported him. Menlo Park was turning into something of a mecca for psyche-delic drug use; some of the key players, alongside James Tyhurst, who attended the Montreal defence summit back in 1951, were starting to conduct research of their own in that corner of California, with the CIA as a silent partner. As early as 1960, the MK-ULTRA program had been conducting tests on volunteers at Stanford University, under the pretense of academic study.

One such volunteer was Ken Kesey. Kesey would turn out to be a critical test subject. A handsome, all-American athlete with a fertile mind, Kesey participated in an LSD trial while working as an orderly at the Menlo Park Psychiatric Hospital, being paid $75 (far better than the $5 offered to test subjects at the University of Saskatche-wan) to sit through an eight-hour acid test. It would change his life. Under the influence of LSD, he realized that hiding behind his good looks and natural athleticism was a young boy, fearful of the world. For the first time, he reflected, he had found real courage, and this newfound confidence helped him overcome the scorn of his creative writing professors (who viewed him as something of a joke) and complete a novel he had been writing: *One Flew Over the Cuckoo's Nest*. Published in 1962, it catapulted him to international fame, and gave him a platform from which he could espouse the gospel of LSD.

Meanwhile, back at Hollywood Hospital, Frank Ogden was working for free.

Having been given a chance to prove himself by Ross MacLean, Ogden sat in on dozens of sessions through 1961 and 1962 — includ-ing at least one with Hubbard — as an unpaid observer. He wasn't the only Hollywood Hospital employee to be hired without a medical degree; another therapist, John Austin, was similarly lacking in aca-demic credentials. Without Hubbard's influence, the sessions assumed a less overtly religious tone, and little by little, the profile of the patients themselves also began to change. In the beginning, those treated were predominantly alcoholics. But as the years passed, patients came seeking psychedelic therapy for any number of reasons.

"His chief reason for undergoing therapy is to attempt to realize more of his creative potential in his chosen field," wrote Dr. D. C. MacDonald of one patient. Another contacted the hospital about wanting "to see in more perspective the relative importance of people, events, and situations" and "to hopefully realize that all problems aren't so urgent as they seem." Yet another wanted to get to the root of his sexual impotence. Regardless of their reasons or their diagnoses, prospective patients all shared a desire for greater self-understanding — one they sought through a clinically supervised dose of LSD. Despite the furious opposition of Tyhurst and the BC College of Physicians, the drug had not yet become a major part of the public conversation.

That was about to change.

By the fall of 1962, Timothy Leary was turning heads — the wrong ones. His experiments at Harvard — always of dubious academic merit — had abandoned all pretense of professionalism. Now, the brash psychologist freely distributed LSD to colleagues, friends, and even his students.

Osmond and Huxley had met Leary back in 1960, on the eve of John F. Kennedy's election, and at the time thought he would make a good advocate for psychedelic medicine.

"I think he's a very nice fellow," he said to Huxley, "but don't you think he's a bit too square?"

Osmond himself would later characterize that assessment as "perhaps the least satisfactory description" of Leary ever made, and by 1962, any early goodwill between them had vanished. In letters, Osmond and Huxley disdainfully referred to Leary as "the Messiah"; the divide between academics and "explorers" (as Osmond called them) was rapidly widening, and the resultant bad publicity risked giving the entire field a black eye.

"So far the explorers are mostly running into trouble, much of it of their own creating," Osmond complained to Huxley in December of that year. "Timothy Leary and his friends seem impervious to the idea that psychedelic substances may be both valuable and dangerous if misused. [...] Timothy Leary has written to me as if he knew all there is to be known about these substances. Dangerously different from the uncertain man we met two years ago. And of course, he is in trouble because he has taken no precautions and could be shot down by anyone who cared to ask the right questions."

And these feelings of resentment only intensified after Leary paid Huxley a visit later in the month, speaking in such outlandish terms about consciousness and authority that Huxley observed it "is the reaction of a mischievous Irish boy to the headmaster of his school."

"I am very fond of Tim," he continued, "but why, oh why, does he have to be such an ass? I have told him repeatedly that the only attitude for a researcher in this ticklish field is that of an anthropologist living in the midst of a tribe of potentially dangerous savages. Go about your business quietly, don't break the taboos or criticize the locally accepted dogmas. Be polite and friendly — and get on with the job."

But their frank assessments paled in comparison to those made by Al Hubbard. Hubbard, a hyperconservative, had become so enraged by Leary's behaviour that during a psilocybin session with Humphry Osmond, he began pondering out-and-out murder.

"Al got greatly preoccupied with the idea that he ought to *shoot* Timothy," Osmond recalled, "and when I began to reason with him that this would be a very bad idea ... I became much concerned that he might shoot *me* ..."

"I think I should say I have never harmed anyone," Hubbard said, recalling his days as a prohibition agent with carte blanche from the government. "I have shot over people's heads, close enough to them — even through their clothes — but I have never harmed anyone. Nor have I had the desire to do so. But should the need arise," he paused, "the capabilities are there."

But Hubbard had his own popularity to worry about.

His lack of discipline, arrogance, and willingness to take unnecessary risks had drawn more attention than usual, alerting Sandoz to the possibility that its LSD samples may have been distributed outside a clinical setting. Albert Hofmann himself wrote to Hollywood Hospital and to the Saskatchewan program to express his concerns. It turns out that, as early as 1959, Hubbard had been playing fast and loose with his supplies, going outside Sandoz's network to amateur chemists and other suppliers whose methods couldn't be verified. Osmond confronted Hubbard, and when he learned the truth, it was the last straw.

By the end of 1962, Osmond, Hoffer, and virtually every reputable academic on the continent had distanced themselves from Alfred M. Hubbard. Sandoz was requiring ever more onerous paperwork to access their samples, and neither Sandoz nor Osmond was willing to provide Hubbard with anything. In a December letter to Huxley, Osmond was outwardly scornful.

"Al Hubbard meanwhile is having his troubles and they are compounding," he wrote. "Al has been ingenious. He has, he believes, outsmarted many of his medical critics, but he forgets that medicine is an old profession and a battle is not a campaign. A campaign is not a war. Al has benefitted large numbers of people — but he has failed to benefit some and may have harmed a few. It has not struck him, so far as I can discover, that his enemies will use this small number of inevitable failures to destroy him. Abram and I have always urged a very different course, getting money for systematic and determined research. Al would not do this so we have learnt all we can from him."

Hubbard, he continued, "doesn't listen to things he doesn't want to hear. Psychedelics are not the answer to everyone's problems, and his ways of using them are not the only way or even the best. Al's notion that hostile medical men only need a slap on the back or a punch below the belt to establish good relationships is mistaken. However we shall have to see what happens."

In 1963, Hubbard's mistake became everyone's problem when Timothy Leary and Richard Alpert were fired from Harvard University.

Rumours flew about the cause of his dismissal — was it related to his psilocybin experiments in prisons? Had he finally crossed the line with his inappropriate sexual relationships? Did his various misdemeanours — drinking and driving, marijuana possession — catch up with him? Or is it that he simply stopped showing up to classes? Whatever the case, news of Leary's dismissal spread across North America, and brought with it renewed scrutiny regarding psychedelic research. Leary retreated to Millbrook, a mansion outside New York City, where his residency as a psychedelic guru brought even more disciples and media attention. Just as Osmond and MacLean had feared, public opinion was souring on psychedelics, and they knew that if they didn't tread carefully, they could find their work at the centre of a full-blown moral panic.

Meanwhile, Frank Ogden was about to embark on some psychedelic research of his own; in May 1963, it was time for his first session in the Acid Room. Settling onto the couch, he ingested a significant amount — 500 milligrams of mescaline and 300 micrograms of LSD — in the presence of therapist John Holloway and Dr. D. C. MacDonald.

For Ogden, the experience was deeply erotic.

First, he found himself transported to the banks of the Nile, surrounded by beautiful naked women.

"These women were full breasted," he later wrote. "Some of their clothing left one breast bare. They were dusky bronze in color with long sinewy legs and healthy sexual appetites. We loved in a million different ways. I was a lusty, healthy pagan. And I loved it."

The visions intensified, and Ogden suddenly felt sick to his stomach. A nurse brought him a bucket and he vomited, removing a sweaty shirt — though he didn't remember perspiring.

"I remember my conscious mind thinking at one point this is a hell of a time to puke," he laughed, "just when you're making love to this pre-Cleopatra Cleopatra on the lush green green green banks of the Nile."

From there, his visions took him through history, past the signing of the Declaration of Independence, to a pirate ship on the high seas. He recalled weeping, thanking the kind doctors for giving him this gift of experience before being again transported away on the notes that filled his mind as music entered his consciousness. He felt as though he was moving through cinematic scenes; he felt the sun on his skin, the wind in his hair, tasted the salty sea air. The music transfixed him, invoking a bright array of scenes and vibrant colours that danced in his mind, conjuring feelings of joy and connection.

"Next and most vivid, I was leading a band of pirate girls, flying the Jolly Roger, conquering all who came in my path," he continued. "The girls again. Dressed so seductively. After a few years of this — or was it a mini-second. I died again. I mean died. I felt the cannon shell tear me to bits, saw the blood, felt the pain, felt the haze and comfort of death."

At this point Dr. MacDonald checked in, asking if he was all right.

"Couldn't he see my pirate crew all around me?" he thought, annoyed. "They were warm, loyal and a great bunch. I recall being annoyed by this petty questioning."

The session continued into the evening, and Ogden was an immediate convert.

"Hooray!" he shouted. "I'm LSD's first addict!"

"But this was so much better a world," he wrote afterward. "Perhaps a world that could be if man could only see all the beauty that existed around him instead of constantly engaging in petty jealousies and bickering."

After the session, he went to the bathroom and "urinated gallons," and was then, in his own estimation, ready to begin his career as Hollywood Hospital's newest therapist. Over the next eight years, Ogden claimed to have worked with over a thousand patients.

"The majority arrived with problems and left as better people," he noted in his later years. "It wasn't always a pleasant experience for them, but nothing worthwhile is."

In many ways, Ogden was a natural successor to Al Hubbard, and he came to perfectly define the new wave of psychedelic explorers, bringing with him a sense of adventure, an open mind, a flair for the dramatic, a total disdain for authority, and no academic expertise whatsoever.

By this point, Al Hubbard's supplies had run out.

Sandoz had recently appointed a committee of investigators to evaluate the scientific legitimacy of each and every request they received, and Hubbard, with his mail-order PhD, didn't qualify. The International Foundation for Advanced Study promptly lost its access, forcing Hubbard to find another avenue. Undeterred, he boarded a plane and flew to Czechoslovakia, where he charmed his way into becoming the North American representative for the LSD being sold by the chemical corporation Chemapol. His new source secured, Hubbard returned to Canada and set up his own psychiatric clinic in downtown Vancouver. As with Hollywood, Hubbard partnered with a legitimate psychiatrist, and placed himself on the payroll as a humble consultant. But the Consera Psychiatric Clinic, as it was known, never measured up to the Menlo Park or New Westminster facilities.

It seemed that the old guard was losing strength.

To Osmond and MacLean's chagrin, new pockets of "explorers" had sprung up everywhere, fed by a mysterious supply of LSD with no discernible source. In San Francisco, Ken Kesey began holding regular "acid tests" with his friends, set to live music provided by his favourite local band, the Grateful Dead. These friends, calling themselves the Merry Pranksters, later staged a bus journey across the country that would be immortalized in Tom Wolfe's seminal work *The Electric Kool-Aid Acid Test*. Contrary to Huxley's plea, Timothy Leary had no intention of keeping quiet and appeasing the authority figures of the day. The rift that had been torn open by Hubbard's visit that fateful day in 1962 now seemed irreparable, the gap between academics and "explorers" too vast to bridge. LSD was no longer simply a research drug for middle-class intellectuals and medical professionals. Against their will, it had been thrust into the court of public opinion, and its future was now under serious threat.

Osmond, MacLean, Huxley, and Hoffer knew they didn't need a messiah.

What they needed was to fight back.

Claire Fisher
October 2, 1964

Claire Fisher came to Hollywood Hospital in search of courage.

Several years earlier, she and her five children had fled the United States and the horrors of her first marriage for Canada. At the time, she wasn't sure she would be up to the task. She was, she wrote, "beset by fears and uncertainty." She worried that she wasn't enough — that she was too broken, too weak, too weighed down by years of trauma.

Then she met Gene. Gradually, he taught her to let down her guard. To find peace. For a short time, he made her believe that she was worthy of love.

"I depended on his strength to keep going," she admitted.

Now he was gone. And she was alone.

Again.

She had lost Gene. She had lost her job. She was about to lose her apartment.

She feared her weakness would ultimately land her in an institution, and had come to Ross MacLean in hopes that a session in the Acid Room might finally "give me a little of the Courage, Strength & stronger Convictions that I lack."

"I know my words are weak," she wrote. "I cannot begin to describe myself or my feelings in regards to LSD, but I know with my whole being that this is something that will help me in many ways. It is one of the biggest desires of my life."

Through psychedelic therapy, she hoped to win Gene back. She hoped for the strength to keep fighting. And she desperately wanted to build a future for herself and her children. But to get to that future, she would need to confront her past.

Her life had been a seemingly endless series of traumas.

Born in Denver, Colorado, as the oldest of three children, she lost her mother at an early age, after complications from a miscarriage.

"I remember my Mother as a happy laughing person," she later wrote. "I remember how she loved to dance and how I would watch her dancing around the room spinning and skirts whirling and her long auburn hair flying. […] She lived as she felt. If she felt like running, she'd run, if she felt like wrestling with us kids in the yard she'd do so."

When Claire was five years old, the family relocated to California. That winter was especially rainy, and they lived in the attic of a rented house, listening to raindrops on the roof, as their father got settled at his new job in Los Angeles.

"I can remember the grey of the days and the constant rain and Mom trying to keep our spirits up and her own as we waited," she wrote. "Our favorite game was laying on the bed and looking at the catalog and picking out the lovely things we would have some day."

Her mother died suddenly. First, there was the miscarriage. Less than a week later, she was dead.

"I didn't believe it possible that my Mother could die," Claire wrote. "It wasn't until I went to the funeral with my Father that I actually knew she wouldn't be coming home anymore. All thru

[sic] the burial the rain poured down in torrents and I thought that God was crying too."

Claire's father joined the navy, sending the children to live with their grandmother, but the burden proved too much, and Claire and her younger sister were subsequently shipped off to a Los Angeles orphanage.

Conditions were grim: the meals were tiny, the rooms were cold, and the discipline was violent. The other orphans were a cruel bunch, and her three-year-old sister became a popular target. By day, Claire found herself fighting off swarms of bullies. By night, they huddled under their blankets with whatever piece of bread or fruit they had managed to steal to fill their aching stomachs.

"We finally earned the respect of the other kids," she wrote, "but I suffered many long hours, and some nights in a dark room with no windows because of my fights."

Refusing to back down, she was branded a troublemaker, and her exile to the windowless room became so frequent she developed a fear of the dark that continued into adulthood.

"I became terrified of the dark because I was even more alone in there," she wrote.

After eight brutal months, they were moved elsewhere. Her brother joined them, and the conditions were marginally better, but the environment had already taken its toll.

"At this orphanage we were visited a few times by prospective parents," she explained. "However I did not want us to be separated and I was suspicious of the people and presented quite a sullen picture. [...] They would often make ado over my petite pretty sister and my little brother who was a beautiful child with a head full of white curls. I remember one woman saying she wouldn't hesitate to take these two, but she certainly wouldn't want me!"

Eventually, her fears were realized — her brother and her sister were both adopted, and Claire was slated for foster care — until her grandmother arrived unexpectedly and, in the dead of night, stole her away.

"We moved from city to city," she remembered. "It seemed like every time we would move in a place we would se [sic] a prowling police car and in fear would move again. I thought this was a grand adventure!! It was a scary exciting time."

They were ultimately apprehended, but, in that short span of time, the bond that formed between grandmother and grand-daughter became too strong to break; her father gave up custody, and for the next four years she lived at her grandmother's home, "loved and spoiled."

But the orphanage years had left more than a few scars.

"I didn't have many friends," she noted. "I had learned to like being alone. I preferred my books, dolls and the peaceful quiet-ness of my grandma's home. We had many wonderful adventures together. We clung together, me needing to be loved and wanted, and my grandmom needing a reason for living and someone to lavish attention on [...] Many's the night my grandma would hold me during the late hours so I would feel safe."

When she was twelve, her father moved back to the US and remarried, and demanded the children return home. But their new life wasn't particularly idyllic.

"[My stepmother] didn't like any display of affection at all," Claire wrote. "When I tried to take my problems to her she couldn't understand them. [...] I still wanted love, and once in a moment of strong emotion I thru [sic] my arms around my stepmother and hugged her, only to have her stand coldly and wait for me to remove my arms."

Adding to her sadness, Claire's grandmother died that same year. Nonetheless, things changed substantially during adolescence. In her teenage years, she blossomed into a beautiful young woman, and suddenly found herself popular with her classmates — boys and girls alike. She also discovered a love of singing, performing in shows and competitions, at functions, and on the radio. At the end of high school, she was awarded a scholarship to the prestigious New York Academy of Music.

Around this time, she met a marine named Bill.

He was handsome, exciting, and attentive, and their courtship proved both swift and intense; in less than a year, they were discussing marriage.

"We were in 7th heaven — the world was ours," she said.

Her parents weren't quite so enthusiastic. Nonetheless, she abandoned the New York Academy and threw herself into married life.

"Our first year was unbelievably happy," she said. "We did everything together. When he came home at night from work he would come running up the stairs to our apartment and find me and swing me around in his arms. And my whole day was spent in planning for and dreaming of him."

Shortly afterward, their daughter Rachel (Charlie) was born; she had a slight deformity in her legs, but the new parents were nonetheless "wild with joy and pride." After Charlie's birth, Claire began to notice subtle changes in her husband. At first, she shrugged it off. Then, they got pregnant for a second time — with twins — and things got substantially worse.

Bill's behaviour became ugly, paranoid. He accused his wife of putting ground glass in his food. He lost his job. The bills piled up, and they were forced to move. At the same time, Charlie's deformity worsened to the point that she had to be fitted with leg braces, and the twins, born prematurely, required round-the-clock care. By then, Bill was unable to work at all, and Claire had to support the family with a succession of odd jobs — hustling as a cocktail waitress, running a dice game, working as a camera girl in a club. On Saturdays, she modelled for a photographer.

"Oddly enough throughout this period I was able to keep my morals high," she chuckled, "even in the surroundings I was in and some of the tempting offers I had!"

Hoping that a change of scene might help, she moved the family to Moses Lake, Washington. But supporting them on a single income proved impossible. They regularly went days without eating. At one point, they were forced to move into a refurbished chicken coop. When they did finally move into a house, the heating barely worked; each morning, they awoke to a kitchen sink full of ice.

"I use [sic] to be afraid to go into the children's room in the morning if they weren't crying," she recalled, "because I was afraid they would be dead."

And as time went on, Bill's behaviour got increasingly bizarre — and increasingly violent.

"Bill started doing things he couldn't remember later," she wrote. "Like waking up in the middle of the night choking me, or throwing me out of the bed or beating me. I was afraid to go to bed at night."

Matters came to a head after he pulled their youngest daughter from her playpen, threw her to the ground, and stomped on her. Without thinking, Claire jumped into the fray — and suffered the consequences.

"He went completely out of his mind and beat me until I passed out," she recalled, "and then went running out of the house."

Bill returned several hours later, with no memory of the incident. Horrified, he called the police, and when they arrived, they took him into custody. Shortly afterward, the state psychiatrist handed down a diagnosis of schizophrenia. Bill was remanded to psychiatric care, and Claire took her family to Ellensburg, a quiet community where she had spent her high-school years. By this time, she was pregnant again, and when Bill was released from confinement, he rejoined the family.

"He seemed to be the old wonderful Bill that I knew before with love in his eyes and full of kindness," she said. "He got a good job, and about two months before the baby was born I went back to him and things were good again. We wanted a son so badly. Bill was the last son in his family and he wanted his family line to go on."

But that son — Louis — didn't survive. And soon afterward, Bill's dark moods returned. So Claire did the only thing she could: she left. She moved to Canada, took a job in a dance studio, and found a cozy home to raise her children. She progressed so quickly at work that she began teaching classes of her own, and fell in with a new group of friends.

"It was a wild fast exciting time," she said. "I started going around with a crowd of rich young people and it was party after party. But after awhile I seemed to be on a merry-go-round. I kept feeling that there must be more to life."

Then she met Gene.

"After I started dating him I realized that he wasn't the average sort of fellow," she wrote. "There was something deeper in him that I was drawn to. I often had the feeling that this was what I had been waiting for, that thru [sic] him I was going to find something I was searching for."

Together, they moved to the remote northern town of Bella Coola, on the northern coast of British Columbia, where Claire began seeing a doctor in hopes of sorting through her trauma. Then, without warning, after five years, Gene walked out. Several weeks later, she lost her job. Then she received an eviction notice. This was, Claire suspected, all her fault. Perhaps those parents at the orphanage all those years ago had been right after all: she was incapable of loving or being loved.

When she arrived at Hollywood Hospital, she was, in her own words, "at a crossroads."

During her intake, the physician in charge remarked, with a total lack of professionalism, that her physical beauty "left a distinct impression," and recommended her as a candidate for psychedelic therapy. The following morning, attended by Ross MacLean, D. C. MacDonald, and Frank Ogden, she was given 500 milligrams of mescaline.

"It seemed like a long time before anything happened at all," she later wrote. "I first noticed sound — the loudness of it, when I ran my finger over the chain on my neck, I could hear it, it startled me — I rubbed my fingers together and then my feet — a great delight seized me and I thought — I'm stereophonic and burst into a million pieces of reds, crimsons and purples."

Lying on the couch with her eyes covered, she saw herself in the middle of a violent storm. She pushed through the gale-force winds, only to land in a dark room. But, unlike the dark rooms of her childhood, this one was soft, warm, and comforting.

"I longed to remain there," she wrote.

Instead, there was a glare of light. Pain wracked her body, and she felt herself falling as if she had been torn from the womb, an "ugly, throbbing red wound" on the floor. She screamed as crowds of people walked on top of her. She tried to move, to sit up, but she was in agony. She felt the pain of childbirth, of physical abuse, of crucifixion.

Then it stopped, and she was a child again, running her hands through her mother's hair as they looked through a catalogue, dreaming of what they would buy when they got to Los Angeles. She saw scenes from her childhood — her mother on her deathbed, a long parade of orphanages and convents, vivid scenes of monstrous orphans.

"Gene, help me, please," she pleaded.

Gene appeared at the edge of her vision, but rather than ease her pain, he simply told her to pray. Then, before her eyes, she saw a heavy, black knotted whip.

"Take this," she cried. "Beat me. This I can stand, but please don't torture my mind anymore. It's too much."

In that moment, she felt desperately alone, and longed for someone to hold her hand.

"I'll hold your hand," someone replied. "I can't help you — you have to suffer this — but I'll hold your hand so you won't be alone."

She couldn't identify the voice. It sounded like nobody she had ever heard. Was it her mother? Gene? Then a cool hand closed around hers, and her grandmother stepped into the light. She wore a floral dress, and a smile danced across her lips. Hand in hand, they walked into a grey hospital room, one that was seeing the first light of sunrise.

"As I turned, a nurse walked silently into the room and handed me the body of my dead son Louis," she wrote. "This was my first son. I felt myself in the same anguish and despair I had felt then. It was real and raw."

Then the walls fell away, and she found herself transported to a graveyard on a sun-drenched hilltop, "looking young and beautiful with my arms full of lovely flowers. As I stood there with a breaking heart, a well meaning woman approached me and innocently said 'My dear, how beautiful you are, you look like a bride.'"

Again, Gene appeared at her side. Again, he urged her to pray. But when she spoke, the words sounded hollow.

So instead, lying on the couch at Hollywood Hospital, she began to sing.

"I found my whole body and soul pouring itself into the words and music," she explained. "I felt the strain, I was singing with my fullest richest peak, with all my heart. I was filled with a feeling of fulfillment and joy, as though I were bursting inside myself."

The song lifted her up into the clouds, down into a deep, black pit, and back out again. As she rose once more into the sky, she begged Gene to join her. He didn't. And as she watched him vanish below, she felt herself transformed.

"I was an amazon of a woman," she marvelled, "huge and golden like a goddess out of mythology."

She caught sight of therapist Frank Ogden and struck out, hurling thunderbolts. A mighty battle ensued, but Ogden "gave me back lightning bolt for lightning bolt and thunder storm for thunder. The heavens whirled with our battle and the earth shook and he won. I collapsed in amusement."

As the music changed to African drums, her newfound power turned sensual. At first, she fought it, shouting at Ogden that it "wasn't fair to look inside me and pull these things out." Then she gave in to the rhythm, and danced with mad abandon. Stars and planets whirled around her, in magnificent shapes and colours. And for the first time since the session started, she didn't feel alone.

"There was a contented feeling of finally being joined, (but I am not sure by whom)," she wrote.

She found out a moment later. Gently, Ogden told her to remove her face mask and handed her a mirror. At first, she refused to look — but only at first.

"I saw many things," she wrote, when she gazed upon her face. "Mary Magdalene — peace — goodness."

Her features shifted and twisted, and for an instant she was afraid, but Ogden urged her not to look away.

"I calmed myself and saw only a shadow of a cross on my face," she wrote, "and then, just my face — and I realized that perhaps I wasn't so bad at all."

She began to cry.

Because in that instant, she knew that she was enough — more than enough. She didn't need Hollywood Hospital to bring her courage. She didn't need Gene to give her strength. She already had both in abundance. Courage had brought her through the orphanage, where she faced down her sister's tormentors and the cruel whims of the staff. Strength had saved the life of their young daughter.

She was more than just worthy of love. She was a warrior, an Amazon, a goddess sheathed in gold, willing to step up and fight when nobody else would. And that Amazon, who had been in so many other people's corners during all those years, was now in her own, and she would never feel alone again.

"I look good," she said through tears. "I didn't ever think I would look good again."

Over the next five years, she stayed in touch with Ross MacLean and Frank Ogden. She sent them cards at Christmas and Halloween, and then, in September 1965, an invitation to her wedding. She had, it seems, moved on from Gene, and the lessons learned from her session in the Acid Room helped prepare her for the battles to come.

They were formidable indeed.

In 1969, Charlie — then fourteen — was taken advantage of by an older man in Bella Coola. Even worse, she became pregnant. Unable to cope with the impending scandal, Claire's new husband threatened divorce. Charlie herself became despondent, talking of suicide. For Charlie's mental health, abortion was the only choice. But the doctor in Bella Coola was a deeply religious man, and abortion was still illegal in Canada unless a committee of doctors agreed that the birth would endanger a woman's life or health.

So, as always, Claire Fisher jumped into the fray.

First, she contacted Ross MacLean. A psychiatric assessment was required to continue the process, and, trying to keep the shameful secret from getting out in Bella Coola, she sent Charlie to the one place she trusted more than any other.

The historical record doesn't reflect how this challenge was ultimately met and overcome — only that it was. Somehow, Claire convinced a medical board to allow the procedure (it's only suggested in the correspondence, but likely because she told them childbirth could trigger a psychotic episode in Charlie, as it had in her ex-husband). She had fought one last battle and won. And after that, she seems to have finally found peace.

Her final correspondence with Ross MacLean was in the form of a Christmas card. It's undated, but appears to have been sent several months after the trouble with Charlie had settled. The card is addressed to MacLean, from both Claire and her husband.

"Dear Ross," she wrote, "Finally & completely — life has been wonderful for me! My happiness knows no bounds! Thanks so much, again, for helping me over the rough spots. Love, Claire."

7

THE GREAT GIG IN THE SKY

Are those lights living? Are they alive with a mind like mine! Or are they lifeless like the moon, just globs and dots of matter without mind or direction. Yes, the answer is obvious. They're lifeless and yet just as beautiful as living things. Life and death are equally beautiful. […] Yes, there's a place for suicide. I'm not ready for it now, for there's too many things for me to live for.

— Gonzalo C., Hollywood Hospital patient, summer 1969

ON NOVEMBER 22, 1963 — the same day as John F. Kennedy's assassination — Aldous Huxley died of metastatic laryngeal cancer at his home in California. Unable to speak and knowing that death was near, Huxley feebly scribbled a note to his wife Laura: LSD, 100 mcg, intramuscular.

She obliged, and Huxley's last few hours on earth were spent peacefully floating in the psychedelic realm, somewhere between heaven and hell. He was sixty-nine years old. To pay tribute to their friend, Humphry Osmond, Abram Hoffer, Al Hubbard, Myron Stolaroff, and others gathered together for an LSD trip. But his death had struck a decisive blow against Osmond, MacLean, and their contemporaries. Though he wasn't a medical professional, Huxley's voice had been a distinguished one, and it lent their work the legitimacy it needed to compete with the likes of Ken Kesey, Timothy Leary, and Hubbard. It took a particular toll on Osmond; Huxley had become a father figure to him, helping to nurture and protect the psychedelic legacy. But now Osmond and the others were on their own.

So they fought back the only way they knew how: with data. In 1965, Ross MacLean and the Hollywood Hospital team published the results of their LSD trials. Entitled LSD-25 and Mescaline as Therapeutic Adjuvants, it was the result of seven years of study and demonstrated remarkable results, showing that half of their patients across most categories showed marked improvements. The most dramatic improvements were in areas of alcoholism, where follow-ups even after fifty-five months showed sustained levels of abstinence for more than fifty percent of patients treated. That May, they presented their work at the second annual International Conference on the Use of Psychedelics in Therapy in Amityville, New York. The paper was politely received in academic circles, but in the outside world, attitudes were changing fast. Throughout 1964 and 1965, the mansion headquarters of Timothy Leary's Castalia Foundation was regularly raided by a zealous district attorney named G. Gordon Liddy (who later achieved infamy as the most incompetent of the Watergate burglars). Ken Kesey too found himself the target of law enforcement harassment, eventually faking his own death and escaping to Mexico.

A series of US Senate subcommittee meetings were convened to address the issue of psychedelic drug use, and when Leary was called as an expert witness, he backtracked on some of his more radical assertions in hopes of staving off prohibition. Legislation, he argued, should require LSD to be provided by licensed, trained adults "for serious purposes, such as spiritual growth, pursuit of knowledge, or their own personal development."

It was too late.

In March 1966, the state of California made LSD possession illegal. Though Canada hadn't yet followed suit, MacLean, Osmond, and Hoffer were nervous. For Osmond, "psychedelic" — the substance and the word he had invented to describe it — was taking on a life of its own; it was now poised to transform not just psychiatry, but North American culture in ways that Osmond found uncomfortable. In March 1967, to Ross MacLean's chagrin, Vancouver's public health officer, J. L. Gayton, published a screed against LSD in the local newspapers — one backed up by the Narcotics Association of British Columbia. The piece made a number of inflammatory — and untrue — assertions, including that LSD could lead to suicide, and that it "shrunk the brain."

So, MacLean and his colleagues went on the offensive.

Several Hollywood therapists, such as Frank Ogden, spoke at community centres and public forums, giving presentations on the safe use of LSD. MacLean, along with Osmond, Hoffer, and others, created the International Association For Psychodelytic Therapy, and began sending out their own press releases.

"Pharmaceutical d-LSD-25 is not addicting [sic]," read one of them. "It is not physically harmful; causes no 'brain damage', nor other organic damage, and no death has been attributed to the drug per se. When competently and ethically used, the likelihood of precipitating prolonged depression, anxiety states or psychoses is of such rarity as to be almost non-existent."

They wrote to the federal government, and to politicians like Tommy Douglas and Senator Robert Kennedy. They matched misinformation with facts, noting, in the case of the much-discussed "acid flashback," that "spontaneous recurrence of perceptual distortions as proof of permanent brain damage is ludicrous [...] the credibility and effectiveness of all warnings is called into question by such overzealous exaggeration."

"We can take a hardline with the authorities," added Osmond. "They have not consulted us. They have acted rashly and things look as if they are going badly and likely to go worse. Young people don't believe their lies and are consequently liable to disregard the truth at the same time to their detriment."

The entire situation, he lamented, was going to result in "the government and professionals looking stupid."

In an open letter, Saskatchewan researcher D. G. Poole added that "those who demanded the prohibition of psychedelics, and those who made the law, were, as has been pointed out, not qualified by their own experience to decide whether these agents are good for people or bad for them."

The current legislation, an exasperated Ross MacLean wrote to a friend, "is a classic example of 'throwing out the baby with the bathwater'!"

But their academic backgrounds made them ill-suited for the fight. The battle was one of feelings — paranoia, revulsion, unease at the inability to control the younger generation. In the meantime, Osmond decided to take matters into his own hands. Seeking to track the source of the underground LSD supply, he went to San Francisco to track down a young man who called himself "the alchemist." His real name was Owsley Stanley, and he was a soundman for the Grateful Dead.

He also happened to be pretty good at chemistry.

Stanley, who did not at first reveal his identity to Osmond, did ultimately invite the psychiatrist to meet with him, explaining that he had figured out how to synthesize high-quality LSD, along with twenty or thirty other chemical compounds that appealed to "Dead Heads." With ready access to Grateful Dead followers, Stanley had distributed millions of tabs of blotter acid, free of charge, and hoped to "change society for the better and to save mankind from the danger of the bomb and from the dangers of a mechanistic and inhuman conformism."

"The huge power of these substances," Stanley claimed, would result "in a semi-political movement that would arise from the commonality of the experience which they can impart — the sense of sharing similar worlds and goals and of being part of a larger whole in a way in which no amount of meetings can do."

Osmond was sympathetic. He came away from the meeting thinking that Stanley was "an ethical man who wishes to better society by molding it to his particular notions." But whatever Stanley's intentions, his supply, and the others springing up around North America, posed serious risks for the work of serious psychedelic science.

Back in Vancouver, increasingly hysterical reports about LSD users were springing up in the media, championed by a UBC neuroscientist and MLA named Pat McGeer. Never one to mince words — even if they were the wrong ones — McGeer was a lauded researcher, and one of a Vancouver Aquarium team that had captured the world's first live orca back in 1964 (and then accidentally killed it several months later, because of a lack of understanding about its physiology). McGeer was also a staunch libertarian, with strong views about individual freedom. This freedom, it seems, didn't extend to drug use; in March 1967, he began urging the BC government to enact a law banning the drug.

"This dangerous drug, contrary to the opinions of some pseudo-experts, does not expand the mind but shrinks it," he claimed, incorrectly, in an April edition of the *Province*. "LSD induces mental illness, and 50 pounds of it can cause mental illness in every person living on the North American continent. It is colourless, tasteless, and extremely powerful, which is why it has been considered for chemical warfare."

Without evidence, McGeer went on to attribute at least two recent suicides to use of the drug, and claimed, baselessly, that it could "lead to addiction which is every bit as hellish as heroin addiction."

Never one to shy away from taking a shot at the city's youth, Vancouver mayor Tom Campbell echoed McGeer's sentiments, urging police to begin frisking young people on the street without probable cause.

"I think the police are making the proper approach in attempting to stamp out the use of these drugs," he told the *Province*. "I think society is entitled to use everything available to it to stamp out this cancerous growth."

Across North America, newspaper reports implicated acid in cases of murder, suicide, birth defects, and all manner of outrageous behaviours.

"LSD Reaching Epidemic Proportions!" shouted a headline in the *Province*.

"Baby Given LSD!" screamed another.

In Philadelphia, a newspaper reported that six students had gone blind after taking LSD and staring into the sun (the official who made the assertion later admitted to lying about the incident, and was consequently dismissed from his job). Drug users, the papers warned, became increasingly detached from society and reality, taking Timothy Leary's slogan "Turn on, tune in, drop out" to dangerous new heights. Absent from comment in any of these articles were Humphry Osmond, Abram Hoffer, or J. Ross MacLean.

There were some who managed to speak out against the mounting moral panic; during a 1967 visit to Vancouver, noted philosopher Alan Watts derided the establishment's zeal for prohibition, urging instead a robust program of public education.

"Police are overburdened people who should be controlling the traffic, preventing robberies, and protecting citizens from violence," he told a reporter. "The police are forced into the function of armed clergymen going around enforcing matters of private morals in the name of the law."

At a public forum, UBC psychologist Robert Halliday spoke in front of 400 people, noting that "little purpose is served by moralizing about marijuana, LSD, and other drugs. The drugs themselves are neither good nor bad."

At the same time, someone else at UBC was looking to dispel the myths around LSD and its users. Her name was Carol Chertkow. A graduate student in the university's department of psychology, she sought to better understand Vancouver's drug users — particularly those in the so-called "subculture" along Kitsilano's Fourth Avenue, a street colloquially known as "Acid Row." Between January and August 1967, she interviewed dozens of Vancouverites and conducted surveys to test how LSD affected their creativity and political views. Her study was divided into two parts, and concentrated on people who fell into four categories: Hippies/beatniks, academics, artists, and "Secret Heads" (business and professional people who didn't advertise their drug use).

Surprisingly, her thesis supervisor was James Tyhurst.

Nonetheless, Chertkow set out to interview as many subjects as possible, and her research stood in stark contrast to the public hysteria surrounding psychedelic drug use.

"A recurrent theme among subjects in both groups [control and experimental] was the characterization of the student-user as a person who is dissatisfied with society and/or himself," she wrote, "and as one who is searching for something to believe in."

LSD use showed no meaningful correlation with antisocial behaviour, but the subjects who had taken it did report "that the LSD experience had changed them in some way."

To better understand her subjects, Chertkow embedded herself with a contingent of Kitsilano hippies. This phase of her research went beyond questions about acid and exposed her to an entire underworld of drugs. To her surprise, she found that LSD users were among the most cautious (especially compared with heroin or methamphetamine users); most of the people she encountered felt that LSD was not dangerous. There were many reasons to question political values, they explained, and taking drugs hadn't inspired these critical views in the first place.

"These people are responding in a particular way to the dissatisfaction and aimlessness which young people in general are feeling," she wrote.

In fact, she found that her subjects tended to share information with one another about how to get the most out of an experience and avoid negative outcomes. This local knowledge was completely discounted by authorities, including Tyhurst and McGeer, and ultimately, studies like Chertkow's were powerless against the mounting pressure to outlaw psychedelics.

Despite the pressure, LSD and mescaline weren't illegal yet, so Hollywood Hospital carried on.

By 1967, the sliding scale for LSD-25 treatment was standardized: $450 CAD for the first treatment, and $250 for each subsequent treatment. Patients were also expected to spend five to seven days in the hospital, at a cost of $18.80 per day. But the number of alcoholics in its patient population had dwindled, to be replaced by more and more people seeking insight.

Later that same year, the BC legislature attempted to pass a law making LSD possession a criminal offence. Owing to the fact that criminal law is a matter of federal jurisdiction, it was passed off to the federal courts, to be examined at the end of 1968. But the likely outcome was clear. Panicked, Hubbard begged Abram Hoffer to let him hide his supply in Hoffer's Canadian Psychiatric Facility in Saskatoon, but Hoffer refused. According to some rumours, Hubbard buried his remaining LSD in California's Death Valley. His supplies gone, his compatriots turning their backs on him, and his finances in ruins, Hubbard was forced to sell Dayman Island in 1968. He and Rita left for California, never to return; he was last seen loading up his boat with the various electronic devices he had collected over the years and stored in his island workshop, the original Acid Room.

Ultimately, the federal/provincial jurisdiction issue had bought MacLean some time. But then, in October, the two final nails were put in the psychedelic coffin.

In BC, Pat McGeer was elected the leader of the provincial Liberal Party, giving him a new pulpit from which to rail against the evils of mind-altering drugs. And south of the border, President Lyndon Johnson signed the federal Drug Control Abuse Amendment, which declared LSD a Schedule 1 substance; simple possession was deemed a felony, punishable by fifteen years in prison. According to Humphry Osmond, Hubbard had lobbied Vice-President Hubert Humphrey, who reportedly took the cause of LSD into the US Senate. It didn't work, and on the advice of the United Nations, Canada followed suit.

Tyhurst, McGeer, and their allies, it seemed, had won. Throughout 1968 and 1969, the papers were filled with lurid stories of teenage drug busts, ruined youth, and hippie LSD cults.

Consequently, psychedelic psychiatry sessions at Hollywood Hospital slowed to virtually zero. For reasons that aren't clear, several more took place, with the last recorded as late as May 1971. The hospital itself continued treating patients until 1975, when the withdrawal of its provincial subsidy, and the generally decrepit nature of the buildings, brought it under fire from the federal government. In the same year, Ross MacLean was sued by a former patient for more than $300,000, alleging undue coercion and medical malfeasance. His legal and financial troubles mounting, MacLean sold the building and cashed out.

Hollywood Hospital's treatment programs, MacLean remarked bitterly in an interview, had suffered from years of "government indifference, obstruction, and bureaucratic myopia."

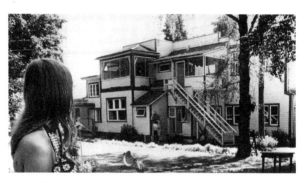

Hollywood Hospital, shortly before its demolition in 1975.
Image courtesy of Postmedia.

When the facility shut its doors in mid-July, Frank Ogden took custody of more than 500 patient files, storing them on his houseboat in False Creek. How or why he came to have them in his possession is unknown, but his intent was clear: to sell the patient info within for a tidy sum. Contained among the patient descriptions, correspondence, therapist assessments, and thousands of pages of deeply personal stories is a letter that arrived in 1971. By then, the Acid Rooms had largely been shut down or repurposed, but, like the hundreds treated there over the years, the experience had stayed with the patient, and he wanted to express his thanks.

"I am still understanding more about my first experience of 67," he wrote. "At that time, I was all set to tell everybody I know about this wonderfull [sic] method of enlightenment, but after telling it to a few, I observed that those who never had a trip couldn't begin to understand, and even those who did have, experienced some thing [sic] unique to themselves, and didn't neccessarily [sic] share my enthusiasm about its potential."

However, he continued, "I still would heartily recommend that everyone takes at least one trip in their life-time. I think I would recommend a minimum age though, because it seems that to get something out of it, it is necessary to have had the opportunity to think about what life is about. All in all, it opens up a lot of very, very interesting avenues in life [...] it was incomparable, and quite unspeakable."

J. Ross MacLean sold Hollywood Hospital for $1.65 million.

In subsequent years, he turned his attention to charitable giving and his membership in the Shriners, becoming the potentate (leader) of his local temple, and eventually head of a national chapter. He sponsored a women's softball team (named Doc's Blues, after him). He bought an island fishing resort and served as director of the Pacific Ballet Company. He also maintained an active interest in the nearly two dozen businesses where he served as director or officer. But his fortunes took a turn for the worse; in 1977, he put Casa Mia on the market, and auctioned off much of the family's furniture. In 1983, his son Stuart died at just thirty-four years old. In 1985, he filed for bankruptcy. His surviving son — a record producer also named Ross — had such severe health problems that he went blind and required a kidney transplant. In his later years, J. Ross MacLean relocated to the Vancouver Island community of Duncan.

He died in 1998.

"Ross MacLean worked hard and played hard," his obituary read. "He was a well of strength and optimism, which those around him drew from often [...] Ross MacLean led a full and meaningful life of service to others. He was a powerful and successful man; a deeply religious man; a loving and generous man; and in his latter years he overcame his adversities with his wonderful sense of humour."

Al Hubbard and Timothy Leary eventually buried the hatchet. In 1979, Leary hosted an "acid reunion," bringing together the psyche-delic pioneers of the '50s and '60s — including Osmond, Myron Stolaroff, Aldous Huxley's wife Laura, and Hubbard. The evening was recorded on video, as the academics and the explorers sat side by side and spoke fondly of the old days. When asked by the camer-aman about his hopes for the future, Hubbard smiled.

"You're the future," he said.

The Captain spent his final years in semi-retirement, in an apart-ment in Menlo Park, attempting to appeal to the FDA for an exemption to continue his psychedelic experiments (this time on end-stage cancer patients). But his health was failing. With an enlarged heart and very little money to carry on, he lived out his final days in a trailer in Arizona, finally forced to stop running. He died in August 1982, at the age of 81.

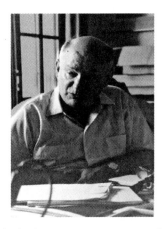

Al Hubbard in his later years. Image courtesy of Fee Blackburn.

Province journalist Ben Metcalfe went on to become an avid environmentalist. Disturbed by the proliferation of nuclear weapons, he boarded a ship called the *Phyllis Cormack*, and set out from Vancouver with a group of young idealists intent on stopping a nuclear bomb test on the island of Amchitka. This group of students and activists would become known as Greenpeace.

In 1989, Dr. James Tyhurst, then professor emeritus of psychiatry at UBC, was accused of sexual assault by four different patients. Their testimony was horrific, involving forced master-slave relationships, non-consensual injections of sedatives, and ritualistic whipping, over a period of more than twenty years. He was found guilty on all counts, and his conviction set off a firestorm in the medical community when it was discovered that his activities had been flagged by the BC College of Physicians as far back as 1981. In civil court, he was forced to pay one of his victims more than half-a-million dollars.

"The nightmare of his 'therapy' will live with her for the rest of her life," wrote Justice David Vickers. "No similar case has been cited to me where the abuse of a care-provider in a position of trust has been so appalling."

American chemist Owsley Stanley is said to have manufactured more than five million doses of LSD throughout his career. Believing a thermal cataclysm was imminent, he moved to Australia, living on a bus in a commune with his partner, and making wearable art. When he died in a car crash in 2011, his cremated remains, as specified in his will, were shot out of a cannon, to serve forever as the Grateful Dead's soundman at their Great Gig in the Sky.

From his houseboat in False Creek, Frank Ogden became a minor celebrity. As a self-described futurist, he travelled the country giving lectures and writing books and newspaper columns about humanity's future potential, even predicting the advent of the Internet. His search for a buyer for the Hollywood Hospital files proved fruitless, however, and he ultimately donated them to the BC Archives. Interviewed about his Hollywood Hospital days in 2007, he reflected back on them fondly.

"They were some of the most interesting and valuable experiences of my life," he said, of his sessions in the Acid Room. "I learned things from LSD, and it still keeps me young in my thinking."

When he died in 2013, he was considered one Canada's best-loved intellectuals.

Albert Hofmann, LSD's progenitor, lived to a startling 102 years of age, still keeping tabs on the field that he had inadvertently pioneered. While he still referred to LSD, famously, as "my problem child," he had grown to accept its utility, even speaking at psychedelic conferences before a new generation of researchers.

Humphry Osmond moved from Princeton to the University of Alabama, where he served as a professor of psychiatry until his retirement in 1992. His research returned to its pre-psychedelic roots, focusing primarily on schizophrenia and psychosis. He worked with Laura Huxley to preserve his letters with Aldous, sensing that their discussions may help future researchers to rediscover the therapeutic benefits of psychedelics; when he died in 2004, his obituary in the *New York Times* called him a "pioneer."

Abram Hoffer left the University of Saskatchewan in 1967 to open a private practice. In 1976, he moved to Victoria, where he more firmly shifted his practice to an interest of his that stretched back to the early 1950s: orthomolecular psychiatry — megavitamins. He is largely remembered today for his promotion of vitamin B and orthomolecular work that also challenged the commercializing forces of psychopharmacology.

Duncan Blewett continued in his position as a psychology professor at the University of Regina. He married one of his graduate students, June, and they retired to Gabriola Island in BC in 1986. He died in 2007, and the Multidisciplinary Association for Psychedelic Studies created a psychedelic research fund in his honour.

Sometime in the early 2000s, Dayman Island found itself under new ownership.

The dilapidated house on the property was in desperate need of renovations, and as crews began their work, stripping it down to the bare bones, they discovered something unusual: hidden behind the drywall was a cache of papers — eighteen pages in all — detailing a series of staff training seminars conducted at Hollywood Hospital in the early months of 1959. Why Al Hubbard chose to stash such an innocuous set of documents inside the walls of his home is unknown; it's hardly salacious, instead serving as a training manual for new personnel, featuring remarks from Hubbard, MacLean, Dr. D. C. MacDonald, and several others. But among the notes on hospital procedure and vitamin regimens was a short meditation on the future of psychedelic medicine, written by a doctor named R. L. Swarovski. It reads more as philosophy than science, and even though it remained hidden away for nearly fifty years, today it stands as a strangely prescient summation of psychedelic medicine, and those who sought to destroy it:

"First, one must assume the premise that man's greatest weakness is his capacity to deceive himself. He starts to gather facts which he believes are real and bases his conclusions on these facts. [...] The word 'knowing' can become a very dangerous thing because it is also a form of deception to man. To know anything by definition is to have an absolute realization of it. There can be no doubt in knowledge; it is absolute in itself and can withstand any type of criticism, philosophical or otherwise. [...] In other words, one may assume that we know nothing but we have only levels of awareness; as soon as one says he knows something he immediately puts up a barrier to his intellectual thoughts and cannot make any further conclusions. [...] If it can be said that man's greatest weakness is his capacity for self-deception then it can also be said that his greatest strength lies in his capacity for re-organizing his weaknesses and doing something about them. It is therefore towards the goal of establishing a higher level of awareness by decreasing the capacity for self-deception that the future of LSD therapy lies. By the intense awareness of a power higher than himself, man can mobilize the courage and effort to face his weakness and do something about them."

The address ends with a rallying cry of sorts, one that wouldn't be answered for decades.

"For the people who are lost, dissatisfied and disillusioned a new avenue of hope is opened," the text continues. "For those who are dying, in pain and agony, the preparation for death with LSD therapy can make all things more tolerable and worthwhile by the understanding gained of the union with a higher power. [...] Certainly all these hopes in a new therapy may seem to be just a dream and I do not wish to suggest it is the answer to all, but I do believe it is the nucleus of a new era of psychiatry — either alone or as an adjunct to other accepted psychiatric procedures or vice versa. Whatever it may be, it is only another stepping stone in our ever constantly changing world of reality."

In September 1975, Hollywood Hospital was bulldozed. Its iconic holly trees were torn up by their roots, and the building's destruction served as a symbolic end to more than a decade of pioneering research into the human mind. After some deliberation by city council, a concrete, two-storey commercial complex was built on the spot, dubbed Westminster Place.

It still stands today, home to two banks, a chain drugstore, and an insurance provider.

ECLIPSE

In 2016, Thomas Hartle was diagnosed with terminal cancer.

His prognosis was grim, and treatment options were limited. In the days that followed, he was crippled by anxiety and depression; he feared for his family, for the future, for his own impending demise and the pain that was to come with it. An IT specialist from Saskatoon, he spent hours on the Internet, and in the course of his research, he stumbled across a Johns Hopkins study indicating psilocybin's use in alleviating depression in end-stage cancer patients. He bought spores online and grew some mushrooms of his own at home. But no therapist would agree to take on his case. Finally, Hartle found Bruce Tobin, a Victoria-based practitioner, and embarked on a psychedelic therapy session.

The results were remarkable.

In a single afternoon, his anxiety score dropped by thirty points. Since Tobin's session, Canada has approved psilocybin for other terminal cancer patients, and they have all reported similar outcomes. After more than fifty years, Canada's attitudes toward drug policy — inside and outside a therapeutic context — appear to be changing. In 2017, Canada's federal government became the first of any G7 country to decriminalize cannabis. Psyche-delics, too, are being re-examined, in Canada and the United States; recent studies have delved into the use of illegal drugs for all manner of mental health challenges, from MDMA for PTSD to ketamine for depression. In 2020, voters in Oregon made their state the first to decriminalize psilocybin for medical use. Other states, including Washington, Florida, and Connecticut, have submitted decriminalization petitions, and cities like Denver, Colorado, have changed municipal orders to allow for the medical use of psilocybin.

And, after decades, Canada is reclaiming its place on the global stage as a trailblazer in the field of psychedelic therapy; in August 2020, Health Canada approved a dozen Section 56 exemptions for the medical use of psilocybin for end-of-life anxiety.

A lot has changed since the prohibition of the late 1960s.

The pioneering figures who are the focus of this book are gone — some, like Leary, Stanley, and Stolaroff, had their ashes catapulted into space. Others, like Osmond and Hoffer, retreated to quieter lifestyles, surrounded by family and adored by patients and colleagues — many of whom had no knowledge of their psychedelic past. As of 2003, Abram Hoffer was still seeing patients on one day per week. Reflecting, he was matter-of-fact about the work he had done with Osmond and the others, musing that society hadn't been quite ready for psychedelic therapy, but that sometime soon those attitudes would change.

It seems he was right.

Prohibition is still in place, and the days of Al Hubbard flying across the country with a briefcase full of LSD are long past, but the approach pioneered by people like him, Ross MacLean, and Humphry Osmond is seeing the light of day for the first time in more than fifty years. Psychedelics are finally being incorporated back into therapeutic environments across North America and Europe. In 2018, journalist Michael Pollan's book *How to Change Your Mind*, about the history and use of psychedelic drugs, shot to the top of the *New York Times* bestseller list. For issues like drug policy, where emotions run high and feelings have historically trumped facts, attitudes will take time to change. And even though a new generation of Canadian researchers stands poised to eclipse the achievements of pioneers like Hubbard, Osmond, and MacLean, the legacy of that lunch meeting at the Vancouver Yacht Club, and the work carried out at Weyburn and Hollywood Hospital, was the first step into a brave new world — one we're only just beginning to fully explore.

ACKNOWLEDGEMENTS

JD:

Thanks, as always, to Mom and Dad, for being the best parents a human person could ask for. Thanks also goes to Brian and Karen at Anvil, for keeping the series going, and for continuing to provide a platform to explore the weird shit. Thanks to Lani Russwurm for the continued back door into newspapers.com (sssssh). To Corey, Emily, Brendan, Amanda, David, Gonz, Cam, Brian, Jesse, Jer, Justina, and Kelly: sorry I used your names. You shouldn't read into it — OR SHOULD YOU? A special shout-out to Hilary Agro, for being such a tireless advocate for harm reduction and common-sense drug policy. You're not afraid to be a warrior, even when it costs you.

Special thanks to Connie MacLean for picking up the phone, and for giving such vivid details of her father and the hospital he ran. Thanks also to Fee Blackburn (Osmond's daughter) for providing photos of some of the key players. Thanks to Brad Holden for unlocking the life of Al Hubbard, and for his unspeakable generosity in providing his manuscript to some guy from Vancouver he didn't know.

A huge thanks to Jess — not only did we survive a bloody pandemic, but we did it while I was jabbering nonstop in your ear about drug policy and dead white guys from fifty years ago. People are boring, but you're something else completely.

And the biggest thanks of all goes to Erika for suggesting we do this thing together. Without you, your insight, and your decades of research, this book would have been about three loose-leaf pages of mediocre details and Pink Floyd lyrics.

ED:

Thanks to Felix and Amelia. You might get sideways looks at the playground when you tell your friends that your mom really loves drugs, but you are amazingly inquisitive little people who inspire me every day. My parents, sisters, niece, and nephews — thanks for always finding ways to make life fun. Thanks to Michael and Cindy Horowitz, for pointing me toward the Al Hubbard papers recovered on Dayman Island. And to my BFF scholar sister Regan, you are awesome; even though you make me exercise, you always make me laugh.

I fell in love with the story of Hollywood Hospital nearly twenty years ago when it popped up on my radar while I was learning about the Saskatchewan psychedelic pioneers. I am grateful to the many people who have helped me to chase down leads on that story: Patrick Barber, Nadine Charabin, Ross Crockford, Raymond Frogner, Brad Holden, Frank Ogden, and Andrew Watson, who helped above and beyond. Thanks to the BC Museum and Archives for granting me access to the incredible records of patients' stories and reports, and special thanks to the many people who helped to transcribe those thousands of pages of handwritten documents: Afsoun Amiraslany, Brandon Brown, Chelsea Clark, Prasenjit Das, Julian Devito-Porter, Chris Elcock, Andrea Ens, Christian Klein, Tarisa Little, Michael Lyons, Forest Onclin, Matthew Oram, Fedir

Razumenko, Lucas Richert, and Blaine Wickham. I really must single out Andrea Ens for her heroic work on this project; she kept us informed and inspired, as she dove into these files and carved out her own incredible analysis of the patients who came seeking conversion and found self-acceptance. Jon Bath at the Digital Research Centre provided much-needed technical support. And, as ever, the support from the Osmond, Hoffer, and Huxley families makes much of this work possible: thanks to Jim Spisak of the Aldous and Laura Huxley Trust Foundation, Fee Blackburn and Julian Osmond, Miriam Hoffer, and Piero Ferrucci.

Since the early 2000s, a lot has changed. What began as an effort to unearth buried stories has become a political topic about transforming mental health services, supporting humanitarian drug policies, and putting Canada back on the map for investing in progressive health care options. Michael Kydd has brought pragmatism and leadership into this space. Thomas Hartle has been the heart of this campaign. Thank you both, and all the others, for bravely pushing this conversation forward.

Jesse, your Pink Floyd lyrics would have joined my unfinished notes on the many stories of the lives that intersected with Hollywood Hospital. Thanks for reaching out. You were the spark that ignited this pandemic publishing partnership. I look forward to meeting in person soon and celebrating our leap of faith. Not just anyone would call up a stranger and end that conversation agreeing to write a book together, then trust that person to share a similar vision for precision and elegance. It was a genuine pleasure.

Patrick Farrell, editor and dear friend: You never doubt me. You read whatever I send you, no matter how ridiculous or last-minute. And you always make things better. Thank you for everything.

APPENDIX A:
AN INCOMPLETE LIST OF
MUSICAL SELECTIONS

"A Perfect Day" (Bing Crosby)

Symphony No. 1 (Mahler)

Nocturnes (Chopin)

"Love's Old Sweet Song" (the Ames Brothers)

"Thy Kingdom Come" (Religious)

"Paul's Letter to the Corinthians" (Religious)

The Rite of Spring (Stravinsky)

Boléro (Ravel)

Concertos Under the Stars (album; Hollywood Bowl Symphony Orchestra)

Brandenburg Concertos (Bach)

"1812 Overture" (Tchaikovsky)

Nocturnes (Debussy)

Symphony No. 9 (Dvořák)

"Lonesome Valley" (Arlo Guthrie)

The Planets (Holst)

Grand Canyon Suite (Grofé)

Hawaiian Shores (album; Webley Edwards)

German Beer Drinking Songs (album; Various)

"Bless This House" (Mahalia Jackson)

"Nobody Knows the Trouble I've Seen" (Mahalia Jackson)

"Lead, Kindly Light" (Religious)

Lure of the Tropics (album; Andre Kostelanetz)

Salome (Strauss)

"South of the Border" (Bing Crosby)

West Side Story (album; Bernstein/Sondheim)

The Moldau (Smetana)

Tristan & Isolde (Wagner)

APPENDIX B:
HOLLYWOOD HOSPITAL:
LSD AUTOBIOGRAPHY

1. State reasons for taking LSD, what you hope to accomplish by it, and the problems confronting you now. Describe birthplace, date, and circumstances surrounding your birth.

2. Discuss early development, temper tantrums, bedwetting, nightmares, illnesses and other unusual feelings or circumstances.

3. FAMILY:
   a) Describe Father — his age; if dead, at what age did he die, and the circumstances of his death. Describe his physical and mental characteristics as a father, husband and person. What was your relationship to him and how did he affect your life.
   b) Mother — Describe as above.
   c) Borthers [sic] and Sisters — Describe similarly.
   d) Any other individuals concerned with your care and development or living in your home.
   e) What effect did you have on your family (i.e.) your family's response to you.

4. EDUCATION: Discuss all aspects of your education, formal education and age accomplished. Describe your attitudes and relationship with teachers and other pupils, and your role in extracurricular activities. Describe your passes and failures, and reasons and feelings re [sic] leaving school. What was our goal in getting an education — if any.

5. ECONOMIC: Discuss jobs held, and your relationship to others at work, your ambitions, successes and frustrations. Number of times promoted or fired.

6. MILITARY HISTORY: Reasons for entering. Age of entry. Service?

Ranks. Promotions, demotions — why? Experiences and attitudes in the Services. Time of, and reason for, discharge.

7. LEGAL HISTORY: Any imprisonments? Charges, fines etc? Reasons for such and results. Attitude to courts, and police. Any other legal involvements such as divorce, law suits, accidents. Describe circumstances and outcome of each.

8. AMBITION: Goals you desire in life.

9. INTERESTS:

10. RELIGION: Describe your religious beliefs, conflicts, concept of God, Heaven and Hell and Death, philosophies, prejudices, and the influence religion and philosophy have on your life. Have you had any religious or mystical experiences?

11. HABITS:
    a) Tobacco — Amount. When started — problems associated with it, etc?
    b) Alcohol — When started, amount, problems associated with it, and how it influences you when under it, and the problem it poses with you, your family and society. Any unusual experiences.
    c) Drugs — Same as with alcohol.

12. SEX AND MARITAL HISTORY:
    a) Describe attitudes developed towards sex, and whence they came. If a woman, describe age of onset of menses, pain associations with it, irregularities. Attitudes, concept of pregnancy, fears, etc., associated with it. Attitudes to change of life, etc.
    b) Describe sexual experiences, circumstances under which they began, with whom, at what age, their age, reasons for it, and feelings associated with it. Describe masturbatory and homo-sexual [sic] experiences, and relationships with the opposite sex. Elaborate on this paragraph only if you wish to.
    c) If married, describe courtship, age of spouse, and reasons and circumstances of marriage, oppositions to it, and conflicts surrounding it. Describe spouse in detail, your relationship with

spouse, attitudes and relationship sexually. Describe attitudes to children, their desirability, their acceptance, ages, and present relationship towards them.

d) Describe all past illnesses and their effect upon you. Describe any fears or phobias, their onset and attitudes towards them. What effect do you think that your ego or personality had on the production of illness? [changes to handwriting] No illnesses of any consequence

e) Discuss any chronic or hereditary illnesses in your family — emotional, alcoholic, other.

13. SELF-DESCRIPTION: What kind of person are you? How do you see yourself as a person? Do you like yourself? Why? Describe your moods, sensitivities, jealousies, adequacies and inadequacies, complexes, fears, guilts [sic], philosophies, capacities for self-deception, your role to other people, your family and yourself. Concept of honesty, sincerity, rejection, etc., — describe in full, etc. What is your ideal of the personality you wish to become. How could you become this ideal?

14. HOW DO YOU FEEL OTHER PEOPLE SEE YOU? Their attitudes towards you, their acceptance of you and their expectations of you, etc.

a) Describe any other outstanding experiences or feelings that have played an important part in your life.

CHAPTER NOTES (BRAIN DAMAGE)

Intro (Speak to Me)

The quote by John Ehrlichman is taken from the April 2016 issue of *Harper's*.

ROYAL VANCOUVER YACHT CLUB, 1953

Details of the meeting between Al Hubbard and Humphry Osmond, and Osmond's recollection of it, are taken from the article "The Original Captain Trips" (*High Times*, November 1991), by Todd Brendan Fahey.

Relevant details about the yacht club itself are taken from *Annals of the Royal Vancouver Yacht Club 1903–1965* (Evergreen Press, 1965).

Further reading on Canada's drug laws can be found in:

Catherine Carstairs, *Jailed for Possession: Illegal Drug Use, Regulation and Power in Canada, 1920–1961* (Toronto: University of Toronto Press, 2006)

Dan Malleck, *When Good Drugs Go Bad: Opium, Medicine, and the Origin of Canada's Drug Laws* (Vancouver: University of British Columbia Press, 2015)

Susan Boyd, *Busted: An Illustrated History of Drug Prohibition in Canada* (Winnipeg: Fernwood Publishing, 2017)

1: Breathe

Further information on Humphry Osmond's theories regarding alcoholism can be found in Erika Dyck's "Hitting Highs at Rock Bottom"

(*Social History of Medicine*, August 2006), and in Dyck's *Psychedelic Psychiatry: LSD from Campus to Clinic* (Johns Hopkins University Press, 2008). On psychiatric transformations, see *Managing Madness: Weyburn Mental Hospital and the Transformation of Psychiatric Care in Canada* (University of Manitoba Press, 2017), by Erika Dyck and Alex Deighton et al.

Further reading on early Swiss investigations with ergot can be found in Beat Bächi's *LSD auf dem Land*.

Albert Hofmann's recollection of the world's first LSD trip is taken from his book *LSD: My Problem Child* (MAPS Publishing, 4th ed., 2017), and the story of Susi Ramstein's tram ride can be found in Erika Dyck and Mariavittoria Mangini's article "Susi's Tram Ride" (*https://chacruna.net/first-woman-to-take-lsd/*).

2: On the Run

Crucial information on the early life of Al Hubbard, as well as several relevant quotes, are taken from Brad Holden's *Seattle Mystic Alfred M. Hubbard: Inventor, Bootlegger and Psychedelic Pioneer* (History Press, 2021).

Duncan Blewett's remark about acid and Al Hubbard's little finger is taken from a 2003 interview with Erika Dyck.

The series of letters between Humphry Osmond and Aldous Huxley was maintained in part by Laura Huxley and Euphemia (Fee) Osmond (Humphry's daughter). Their full correspondence was published in *Psychedelic Prophets* (McGill-Queen's University Press, 2018), and relevant letters in this chapter include: Osmond to Huxley, December 7, 1954; Osmond to Huxley, December 24, 1954; Osmond to Huxley, January 11, 1955; Huxley to Osmond, January 12, 1955; Osmond to Huxley, July 1955; Huxley to Osmond, June 29, 1956; Osmond to Huxley, June 12, 1957; and Hubbard to Hoffer, March 14, 1955.

Osmond's recollection of Hubbard's encounter with the airline pilot is taken from the Provincial Archives of Saskatchewan's (hereafter PAS) Hoffer Collection, PAS, (A207, XVIII. 3b. Osmond to David Lester, August 17, 1956, p. 2, and A297, XVIII. 3b. Osmond to David Lester, August 17, 1956, p. 3).

Hubbard's remarks about the Attorney General of California and the discussion of Hubbard's diploma are both taken from the PAS (A207 109, Letter from Hubbard to Hoffer, February 15, 1956, and SAB A207 109, Letter from Hoffer to Hubbard, January 9, 1956, respectively).

3: Time

J. Ross MacLean's background in harm reduction can be found in the April 19, 1955, issue of the *Province*. Other personal details are taken from his obituary in the *Vancouver Sun*, September 19, 1998.

Ben Metcalfe's descriptions of Al Hubbard and MacLean, as well as all related quotes and recollections, are taken from his article "Doctor Acid" in the April 1980 issue of *Vancouver Magazine*.

Hubbard's remarks about raising money come from two letters to Humphry Osmond (PAS, A207 109, Letter from Hubbard to Hoffer, October 11, 1957, and A207 109, Letter from Hoffer to Hubbard, October 3, 1957). His letter regarding the LSD supply chain can be found at the PAS (Hubbard Osmond Correspondence, October 5, 1958, and A207 1040, Hubbard to Hoffer, November 1, 1958, p. 2, respectively).

Information about the anonymous university professor and all relevant quotes are taken from Al Hubbard's "LSD Session Report: Subject 'University Professor,'" April 17, 1957 (PAS, A207 109).

The letter regarding the Catholic priest's LSD session, dated December 8. 1957, is taken from the New Westminster Archives.

DOUG HEPBURN

Details on the life of Doug Hepburn and all related quotes are taken from three sources: Hollywood Hospital's patient files, the November 21, 1993, edition of the *Vancouver Province*, and the March 25, 1967, edition of the *Vancouver Sun*.

4: Money

The detail about the backwards clock is taken from an author interview with Connie MacLean, August 2021.

James Tyhurst's attendance at the Montreal Waldorf Astoria defence forum is reported in the November 6, 1986, issue of *New Scientist*, and relevant details about his life and career are taken from the September 1, 1991, issue of the *Journal of the Canadian Medical Association*.

Ross MacLean's remarks at the Hollywood Hospital training sessions are courtesy of the Hubbard papers recovered from the walls of his Dayman Island home. They were digitized and donated to Purdue University in 2011 (Hollywood Hospital program and lecture notes, ID # MSP90i001).

Hubbard's remarks about having a "fine group of scientists" can be found in a letter in the PAS (A207 109, Hubbard to Hoffer, February 17, 1959). His complaints about losing interest in science are taken from another letter (PAS A207 109, Letter from Hubbard to Hoffer, October 11, 1957).

5: Any Colour You Like

The anecdote about Andy Williams and Guy Mitchell at Casa Mia is taken from an interview with Connie MacLean, August 2021.

Context on the life of Frank Ogden and his quote about adventure are taken from Jake MacDonald's "Peaking on the Prairies" (*The Walrus*, June 2007).

Ben Metcalfe's report on "the Experience" and all related quotes (including Ross MacLean's) are taken from the August 31 and September 1–5 1959 issues of the *Province*, as well as the April 1980 issue of *Vancouver Magazine*.

Humphry Osmond's letter to Aldous Huxley can be found in *Psychedelic Prophets* (Osmond to Huxley, December 9, 1959).

6: Us and Them

Timothy Leary's quotes about his meeting with Al Hubbard are taken from the 1991 story in *High Times*.

Humphry Osmond's initial assessment of Leary is taken from video recorded during an "acid reunion" of early pioneers that took place at Leary's home in 1979, and has since been made available on the Internet. Those present included Hubbard, Myron Stolaroff, Oscar Janiger, Osmond, and Leary.

Correspondence between Osmond and Aldous Huxley is taken from *Psychedelic Prophets* (Osmond to Huxley, March 7, 1961; Osmond to Huxley, December 18, 1962, Huxley to Osmond, December 26, 1962).

For further reading about Ken Kesey, see Rick Dodgson's *It's All a Kind of Magic: The Young Ken Kesey* (University of Wisconsin, 2013). On Timothy Leary, see Robert Greenfield's *Timothy Leary: A Biography* (Harcourt, 2006) and Don Lattin's *The Harvard Psychedelic Club* (HarperOne, 2011). For background on the Merry Pranksters, see *The Electric Kool-Aid Acid Test*, by Tom Wolfe (New York: Farrar Strauss, and Giroux, 1968).

Anecdotes from Frank Ogden's LSD experience come from notes shared with Erika Dyck in 2006, and from "Patient's Description of Experience (Frank Ogden)" in the Hollywood Hospital patient files.

7: The Great Gig in the Sky

The quote about LSD being not "addicting" comes from a news release by the International Association for Psychodelytic Therapy, March 27, 1967.

D. G. Poole's open letter can be found at the University of Regina Archives (Duncan C. Blewett, 88-29, Box 3, "Others' Writings on Narcotics Legislation," open letter from D. G. Poole, c. 1967).

For further reading on Humphry Osmond's response to prohibition, see:

Erika Dyck, " 'Just Say Know': Criminalizing LSD and the Politics of Psychedelic Expertise, 1961–8," *The Real Dope: Social, Legal, and Historical Perspectives on the Regulation of Drugs in Canada*, edited by Ed Montigny (Toronto: University of Toronto Press, 2017), 169–96.

Carol Chertkow's observations about drug users, and all relevant quotes, are taken from "LSD in Vancouver: A Study of Users" (University of British Columbia, unpublished thesis, 1968).

Ross MacLean's complaints about government myopia at Hollywood Hospital, and the details of its sale, are taken from the July 8, 1975, edition of the *Province*.

Eclipse

Thomas Hartle's recollection of his psychedelic therapy sessions comes from a personal communication with Erika Dyck (May–August 2021).

The entirety of R. L. Swarovski's address at the Hollywood Hospital training seminar is taken from "Hollywood Hospital Program and Lecture Notes" (Purdue University, MSP90i0oi).

ABOUT THE AUTHORS

ERIKA DYCK is a Professor and a Canada Research Chair in the History of Health & Social Justice at the University of Saskatchewan. She is the author of *Psychedelic Psychiatry* (2008); *Facing Eugenics* (2013); co-author of *Managing Madness* (2017), and co-editor of *Psychedelic Prophets* (2018).

JESSE DONALDSON is an author and journalist whose work has appeared in *VICE*, *The Tyee*, *The Calgary Herald*, the *WestEnder*, the *Vancouver Courier*, and many other places. His first book, *This Day In Vancouver*, was a finalist for the Bill Duthie Booksellers' Choice Award (BC Book Prizes). He is also the author of the first two volumes in the 49.2 Series, *Land of Destiny: A History of Vancouver Real Estate*, and *Fool's Gold: The Life and Legacy of Vancouver's Town Fool*. He lives in Vancouver.